LOW BACK PAIN

EDITED BY
LOUIS G. JENIS, MD
CLINICAL ASSISTANT PROFESSOR OF
ORTHOPAEDIC SURGERY
TUFTS UNIVERSITY SCHOOL OF MEDICINE
DEPARTMENT OF ORTHOPAEDIC SURGERY
NEW ENGLAND BAPTIST HOSPITAL
BOSTON, MASSACHUSETTS

SERIES EDITOR
THOMAS R. JOHNSON, MD
ORTHOPAEDIC SURGEONS, PSC
BILLINGS, MONTANA

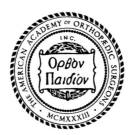

American Academy of Orthopaedic Surgeons

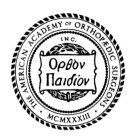

AMERICAN ACADEMY OF ORTHOPAEDIC SURGEONS BOARD OF DIRECTORS, 2005

Low Back Pain

<mark name="0">*Published by*</mark>

American Academy of Orthopaedic Surgeons
6300 N. River Road
Rosemont, IL 60018
1-800-626-6726

The material presented in *Low Back Pain* has been made available by the American Academy of Orthopaedic Surgeons for educational purposes only. This material is not intended to present the only, or necessarily best, methods or procedures for the medical situations discussed, but rather is intended to represent an approach, view, statement, or opinion of the author(s) or producer(s), which may be helpful to others who face similar situations.

Some drugs or medical devices demonstrated in Academy courses or described in Academy print or electronic publications have not been cleared by the Food and Drug Administration (FDA) or have been cleared for specific uses only. The FDA has stated that it is the responsibility of the physician to determine the FDA clearance status of each drug or device he or she wishes to use in clinical practice.

The U.S. FDA has expressed concern about potential serious patient care issues involved with the use of polymethylmethacrylate (PMMA) bone cement in the spine. A physician might insert the PMMA bone cement into vertebrae by various procedures, including vertebroplasty and kyphoplasty.

PMMA bone cement is considered a device for FDA purposes. In October 1999, the FDA reclassified PMMA bone cement as a Class II device for its intended use "in arthroplastic procedures of the hip, knee, and other joints for the fixation of polymer or metallic prosthetic implants to living bone." The use of a device for other than its FDA-cleared indication is an off-label use. Physicians may use a device off-label if they believe, in their best medical judgment, that its use is appropriate for a particular patient (eg, tumors).

The use of PMMA bone cement in the spine is described in Academy educational courses, videotapes, and publications for educational purposes only. As is the Academy's policy regarding all of its educational offerings, the fact that the use of PMMA bone cement in the spine is discussed does not constitute an Academy endorsement of this use.

Furthermore, any statements about commercial products are solely the opinion(s) of the author(s) and do not represent an Academy endorsement or evaluation of these products. These statements may not be used in advertising or for any commercial purpose.

First Edition
Copyright © 2005 by the
American Academy of
Orthopaedic Surgeons

ISBN 0-89203-374-6

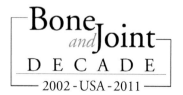

CONTRIBUTORS

Todd J. Albert, MD
Professor and Vice Chairman
Department of Orthopaedics
Thomas Jefferson University Medical College
Philadelphia, Pennsylvania

Howard S. An, MD
Morton International Professor of Orthopaedic
*   Surgery*
Director of the Division of Spine Surgery
Department of Orthopaedic Surgery
Rush Medical College
Rush-Presbyterian-St. Luke's Medical Center
Chicago, Illinois

David Fish, MD
Assistant Professor
Department of Orthopaedic Surgery
David Geffen School of Medicine at UCLA
Los Angeles, California

Carol Hartigan, MD
Assistant Clinical Professor of Rehabilitation
Harvard Medical School
Boston, Massachusetts

Alan S. Hilibrand, MD
Associate Professor
Department of Orthopaedic Surgery
Director
The Rothman Institute South Jersey Spine
*   Center*
Thomas Jefferson University Medical College
Philadelphia, Pennsylvania

Brian Ipsen, MD
Spine Fellow
Tufts University School of Medicine
Department of Orthopaedics
New England Baptist Hospital
Boston, Massachusetts

Louis G. Jenis, MD
Clinical Assistant Professor of Orthopaedic
*   Surgery*
Tufts University School of Medicine
Department of Orthopaedic Surgery
New England Baptist Hospital
Boston, Massachusetts

James Reilly Keffer, DO
Spine Fellow - Physiatry
Department of Physical Medicine and
*   Rehabilitation*
New England Baptist Hospital
Boston, Massachusetts

David Kim, MD
Assistant Professor
Department of Orthopaedic Surgery
Tufts University School of Medicine
New England Baptist Hospital
Boston, Massachusetts

Steven S. Lee, MD
Fellow, Spine Surgery
Department of Orthopaedic Surgery
David Geffen School of Medicine at UCLA
Los Angeles, California

Contributors (cont.)

Sameer Mathur, MD
Fellow, Spine Surgery
Department of Orthopaedic Surgery
Rush Medical College
Rush-Presbyterian-St. Luke's Medical Center
Chicago, Illinois

Anh Quan Quoc Nguyen, DO
Physical Medicine and Rehabilitation Pain
*   Fellow*
Department of Physical Medicine and
*   Rehabilitation*
David Geffen School of Medicine at UCLA
Los Angeles, California

James Rainville, MD
Assistant Clinical Professor
Department of Clinical Medicine and
*   Rehabilitation*
Harvard Medical School
Chief, Physical Medicine and Rehabilitation
New England Baptist Hospital
Boston, Massachusetts

Alexander R. Vaccaro, MD
Professor
Department of Orthopaedic Surgery
Thomas Jefferson University Medical College
Philadelphia, Pennsylvania

Jeffrrey C. Wang, MD
Associate Professor
Department of Orthopaedic Surgery
David Geffen School of Medicine at UCLA
Los Angeles, California

CONTENTS

PREFACE

The spine is a complex structure providing mobility, load bearing capacity, and protection of neurologic components. It also is the source of one of the most disabling symptoms in every person: low back pain (LBP), which is second only to the common cold as a cause for adults seeking medical advice and for work absences in people younger than age 55 years. Up to two thirds of the population will have LBP symptoms at some time in their lives; however, only 14% have an episode lasting longer than 2 weeks, and more than 90% feel better in less than 2 months. During this short period, patients often undertake costly treatments because of the severity of pain and disability. Among those with continuing pain 12 weeks after onset, most still have some symptoms at 1 year. Unfortunately, only 7.4% of patients with LBP account for 75% of the health-care expenditure on back pain.

Although chronic LBP represents a significant epidemiologic and socioeconomic concern, orthopaedic surgeons are just beginning to understand the pathophysiology of the syndrome: how it corresponds to pain perception and disability. An appreciation of the intricacies of lumbar spine anatomy at the structural, macroscopic, and cellular levels is critical to fully understanding the nature of degeneration and pain production. Over the last several decades numerous advances have been made toward management of this chronic disorder. The conventional treatment of chronic LBP has been nonsurgical with standard regimens of medications, exercise, and physical therapy, activity modification, and injection therapy. Surgical arthrodesis remains the "gold standard" for the management of patients who fail to respond to a prolonged nonsurgical program. More recently, alternatives to fusion have become available, with an inestimable number likely to be developed in the future.

Most orthopaedic surgeons deal with chronic LBP on a daily basis, often feeling inundated with reports and studies that do not provide direction in terms of patient care. This monograph was designed with the hope that it will provide a basic understanding of anatomy, pathology, natural history, and treatment options, thereby improving the physician's ability to provide service to patients.

It was not difficult to select topics for this monograph, and I feel fortunate to have been able to recruit leaders in the field of spine care and surgery to assist me in this endeavor. These authors have presented an exemplary review of the current state of chronic LBP pathology, clinical evaluation, and diagnostic and treatment options.

David Kim describes the epidemiology, symptomatology, and differential diagnosis of chronic LBP. James Rainville and associates have written extensively on nonsurgical management of chronic LBP and are considered some of the leading physiatrists in the United

States in the field of nonsurgical care. Jeff Wang, who has contributed a great deal to the literature on lumbar degenerative disorders, covers the various radiographic options and diagnostic injection techniques that form the basis for later discussion of surgical options. Howard An and associates place LBP into a proper perspective when discussing surgery. They discuss numerous surgical approaches to LBP, including anterior, posterior, and combination procedures, as well as reasonable expected outcomes.

In the opening chapter, my former fellow Brian Ipsen and I discuss the normal and degenerative anatomy of the lumbar spine, attempt to relate mechanical changes with biochemical alterations, and discuss the degenerative cascade with reference to potential sources of pain localization. In the last chapter, I discuss some of the new technologies that are currently available or will become available in the future, including artificial disk replacement and dynamic stabilization.

I am truly grateful to my colleagues for contributing to this monograph and appreciate their hard work and timeliness. I would also like to thank the staff of the AAOS Publications Department, especially Joan Abern, Senior Editor, and Lynne Shindoll, Managing Editor, for their assistance in preparing this project and their confidence in me for bringing it to fruition.

So many people have provided assistance that it is nearly impossible to thank everyone; however, I am grateful to my secretarial administrator, Ellen Cohen, for always keeping me on time, and to Kelsey Miller, Research Director, Boston Spine Group, for all her help with writing, formatting, and submitting chapters, figures, and pictures.

Finally, I would like to thank my wife and best friend, Janice, and children, Chris and Tim, for without their understanding of my goals and desires I would not be able to accomplish some of the objectives that I have outlined.

Because it presents state-of-the-art information that will be clinically applicable, general orthopaedic surgeons as well as fellowship-trained spine surgeons, despite varying levels of expertise, will find some important information that they will be able to use to better treatment of the patient.

Louis G. Jenis, MD
Editor

CHAPTER 1

LUMBAR SPINE ANATOMY: STRUCTURE, FUNCTION, AND DEGENERATION

LOUIS G. JENIS, MD
BRIAN IPSEN, MD

An appreciation of the complexities of lumbar spinal anatomy at the structural, macroscopic, and cellular levels is critical to full understanding of the nature of degeneration, pain production, and mechanical function and of the treatment options available to patients with chronic low back pain. The lumbar spine is a unique bony and ligamentous structure that can withstand excessive loads while simultaneously protecting neurologic function and providing flexibility and stability. The intricate interplay between the different anatomic components of the lumbar spine provides efficient motion and function.

MORPHOLOGIC AND FUNCTIONAL ANATOMY OF THE LUMBAR SPINE

The five vertebral bodies and intervertebral disks of the lumbar spine withstand significant physiologic loads, including 1.0 to 2.5 body weights during normal walking and 8 to 10 body weights during lifting of 14- to 27-kg objects.[1] The intervertebral segment of the lumbar spine consists of a three-articulation complex, the disk-vertebral body and two posterior apophyseal (facet) joints, to resist these high loads and stresses. The vertebral bodies are a cylindrical mass of cancellous bone with a cortical shell,[2] and the disks consist of the anulus fibrosus, the nucleus pulposus, and the cartilaginous and bony end plates of the vertebral bodies. The vertebral bodies and disks form the anterior column of the spine, which is responsible for resisting approximately 80% of axial compressive loads and maintaining spinal rigidity and alignment. The intervertebral disk maintains separation of the vertebral bodies and serves as a passive mechanism to distract the anterior column of the spine. The anterior part of the disk is thicker than the posterior part and is responsible for most of the lumbar lordosis because the vertebral bodies are near uniform in shape. Nearly two thirds of lumbar lordosis

FIGURE 1

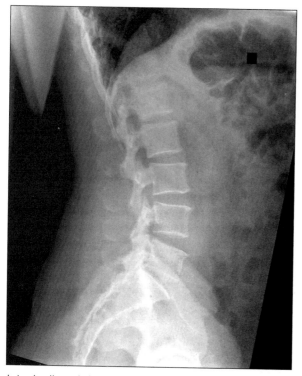

Lateral radiograph depicting normal lumbar anatomy. Note that most lordosis is maintained at the L4-S1 segments.

is localized between the L4 and S1 segments (Figure 1).

The posterior column of the spine consists of the spinous processes, lamina, transverse processes, and facet joints; together, these structures control movement and resist forces. The paired facet joints have hyaline cartilaginous surfaces and are synovial-lined articulations formed by the superior and inferior articular processes of subjacent vertebrae with a fibrous joint capsule. The superior articular process faces posterior and medially, and the inferior articular process faces lateral and anteriorly. The joint surface is oblique to the sagittal plane and facilitates slight flexion and extension or sagittal plane rotation as each articular process glides on the other. The alignment of the facet joints relative to the sagittal plane ranges from 120° to 150°. This orientation resists anterior or posterior translation in normal anatomic alignment and axial rotation in the horizontal plane.[1-4] The bony anatomy serves as a load-bearing structure, a passive restraint to torsional strain and excessive tensioning of the anulus fibrosus, and as a means of protection against disk injury.[5-8]

The posterior column also has ligamentous structures and muscles. The primary functional ligaments of the lumbar spine are the anterior and posterior longitudinal ligaments, interspinous ligaments, and ligamentum flavum, which are oriented longitudinally along the spinal column and resist stretch or principally flexion moments.[9] The iliolumbar ligaments attach to the ilium and L5 vertebra transverse processes, are oriented in a more transverse plane, and act to limit anterior translation and rotation. These ligaments make the lumbosacral junction a very stable articulation.[10-12] The small, multilayered series of paraspinal muscles in the lumbar spine originate and insert on the spinous, transverse, and mammillary processes near the facet joints. Their longitudinal orientation allows them to serve as an active restraint to flexion and possibly to provide proprioceptive sensation during motion. When contracted, these muscles also apply a compression load to the facet joints. The posterior spinal musculature provides minimal restraint to rotation, which is principally compensated for by the oblique musculature.

BIOMECHANICS OF THE INTERVERTEBRAL DISK

Each component of the intervertebral disk has a specific histologic composition and structure that is responsible for a specific function. The vertebral end plates consist of cortical bone in the periphery, which in adolescence is referred to as the ring apophysis, and compressed cancellous bone in the central disk area, which covers nearly 70% of the disk. The outer 30% consists of dense cortical margin and is the strongest area of the end plate. The anulus consists of multiple layers or lamellae of collagen fibers[10-20] arranged in a unique circumferential orientation along the disk periphery. Each lamella is oriented at a 30° angle to the horizontal axis of the disk, and this pattern alternates in successive lamellae.[1] The outer collagen fibers attach to the ring apophysis, and the inner layers attach to the end plate and surround the nucleus (Figure 2).

The annular fiber orientation within the lamellae allows for resistance to tension. The obliquity of the lamellae results in tension or relaxation of the fibers in

FIGURE 2

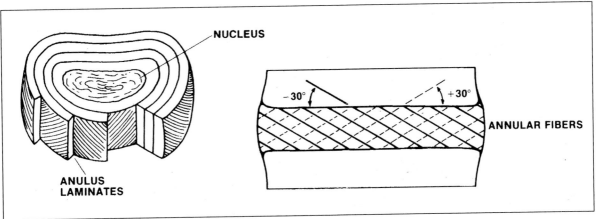

Intervertebral disk structure showing annular fiber orientation and structure. *(Reproduced with permission from White AA III, Panjabi MM: Clinical Biomechanics of the Spine, ed 2. Philadelphia, PA, Lippincott, 1990, p 5.)*

different areas within the disk (anisotropy) and with different forces.[1] For example, in anterior or posterior translation of a vertebral body and disk along the horizontal axis, all of the fibers of the anulus are stretched in the direction of the applied force. However, fibers aligned in the direction of the force (every other lamella) will undergo strain while the remaining fibers actually will be brought closer to one another and will relax. This alternating tension and relaxation with translation and axial rotation maintains the stability of the intervertebral segment.

The nucleus is an incompressible, semifluid composite in the center of the disk space.[1] Under forces of isolated axial compression, the nucleus expands radially toward the inner aspect of the anulus fibers; the anulus fibers also expand circumferentially. Anterior flexion or sagittal plane rotation of the lumbar spine involves a combination of physical events within the disk that exemplify the complex structure and functional aspects of its components. As the vertebral body rotates anteriorly, the anterior anulus is compressed. The nucleus also is compressed eccentrically over its anterior aspect, after which it deforms and migrates posteriorly. The posterior annular fibers expand radially by the shifting nucleus, and the fibers stretched in line with these forces resist further motion. As rotation occurs, the weight of the upper body and trunk lead to shear strain forces at the disk, and slight translation, which is resisted by the

active and passive constraints of the posterior column, may occur.

This interaction of the anterior and posterior lumbar spinal columns is critical for normal physiologic function, load transmission, and kinematics. Lumbar range of motion varies between vertebral levels and individuals. The instantaneous axis of rotation continually changes throughout the range of motion and typically is located posterior to the midvertebral body and below the superior end plate of the inferior vertebral body except at L5-S1, where it is located posterior to the disk space.[13]

CELLULAR BIOLOGY OF THE INTERVERTEBRAL DISK

The cellular and tissue components of the disk include chondrocytes and fibroblastic-type cells in the anulus, nucleus, and end plates that are within an extensive, intricate extracellular matrix (ECM).[13-15] These cells are responsible for homeostasis of the ECM, including matrix formation, maintenance, and remodeling; they derive their nutrition from diffusion across the hyaline cartilage and subcortical end plates; and they flourish within the avascular disk. The cells in the central part of the disk lie closest to the end plate and subsequent vascular supply and are responsible primarily for nutrient and waste product exchange. The ultrastructure of

FIGURE 3

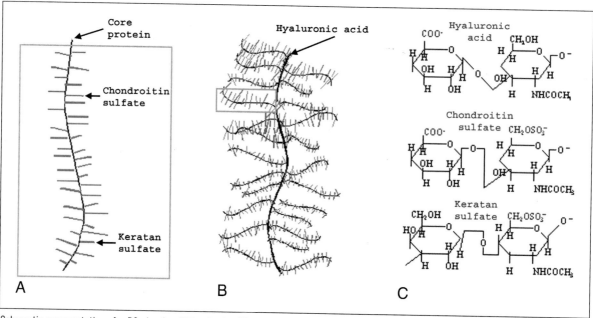

Schematic representation of a PG showing GAG subunits **(A)** and of multiple GAG subunits attached to a hyaluronate filament **(B)**, along with their respective chemical structures **(C)**.

the bony end plate comprises numerous sinusoids with specialized loops of capillaries that come into close contact with the underlying cartilaginous layer. Simple diffusion of molecules across the cartilage is allowed but limited to appropriately sized small nutrients.[16,17] The avascular nature of the disk leads to anaerobic metabolism with a latent acidic pH within the disk under normal conditions.[14]

The cells are responsible for production and constant remodeling of the principal components of the ECM, including collagen and proteoglycans (PG).[14] Collagen provides strength to the disk and is most abundant in the outer anulus; it makes up close to 70% of the dry weight of the anulus but only 20% of the dry weight of the nucleus. Conversely, the greatest concentrations of PG are found in the nucleus (50% of dry weight) and determine the viscoelasticity and stiffness properties of the disk.[14]

The concentric orientation of collagen fiber in the anulus is, as previously described, a series of sheets or lamellae of fibrils, each perpendicular to the adjacent layer. The densely packed layers consist principally of type I collagen, which is highly cross-linked for increased strength, and small amounts of types II, III, V, VI, and XI collagen.[13,14,18] Fibroblasts that diminish in number closer to the disk center are interspersed. The inner anulus contains a relatively greater proportion of chondrocytes and varying amounts of type II collagen fibrils in a loose, nonorganized manner. The central nucleus is a gelatinous core containing chondrocyte-like cells and nearly 85% of type II collagen with some type I, VI, and XI fibers.[14,18]

PGs consist of a protein core covalently attached to a glycosaminoglycan (GAG) subunit (Figure 3, *A*). The GAG units are hydrophilic in nature and retain water in its normal state. Normal water content within the disk is close to 70% to 90%. Chondroitin sulfate and keratan sulfate are the most common GAGs found in the disk, with the former more prevalent in the normal, healthy functioning unit.[14] Multiple PG subunits are attached to a central hyaluronate filament by a glycoprotein known as a link protein (Figure 3, *B* and *C*). The entire structure forms aggregate molecules, of which aggrecan is the largest found in the anulus, although there may be others of variable size and composition including versican, decorin, biglycan, and fibromodulin.[13,18] Fibroblasts and chondrocytes are suspended within this mesh framework along with remnants of notochordal-like cells.

In the normal intervertebral disk, there is a gradient of the cellular and ECM components from the fibrous well-organized periphery to the randomly organized gelatinous center, and these basic molecules provide for well-balanced function (Figure 3). The gradient progresses through four less distinct zones of the disk, specifically the outer anulus, inner anulus, transition zone, and central nucleus. These compounds interact with water to provide the mechanical and structural integrity of the intervertebral disk. The hydrophilic nature of the GAG molecules yields a highly hydrated amorphous central disk structure that in the normal state is constantly under expansible stress. Even when the disk is unloaded, there is a resting baseline intradiskal pressure. The nucleus retains water and expands, providing stiffness and resistance to compressive forces through an interaction of type II collagen fibers and PG. The incompressible nucleus transmits stresses to the anulus where the type I collagen fibers stretch. This mechanism effectively transfers compressive load on the nucleus to a radially directed force with tensile stress to the anulus. Constant load on the disk applies pressure to the nucleus, reducing the ability of the PG and, thus, the nucleus to hold water, causing creep of the disk.[1] As pressure is steadied or relieved, the time-dependent viscoelastic properties of the disk nucleus allow it to regain water.

PATHOGENESIS OF DISK DEGENERATION

Cellular and Biochemical Changes of Spondylosis

The development of lumbar degeneration or spondylosis is ubiquitous and can be seen on the biochemical, cellular, and morphologic levels.[19] The initial events of disk degeneration are related to many intrinsic and extrinsic factors, including cellular apoptosis or programmed cell death, mechanical disk injury, and genetic contributions.[14,18,20-30]

The seminal event likely is related to compromised

FIGURE 4

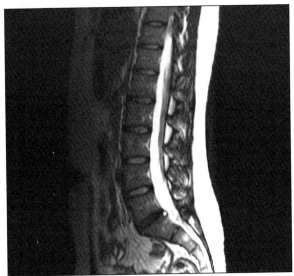

Sagittal MRI scan showing early degenerative changes indicated by loss of hydration and "dark disk" development at L5-S1.

nutrient diffusion and disk hydration[18,31] (Figure 4). End-plate porosity is reduced as a result of subchondral sclerosis and an impaired vascular supply, with shrinkage of pore sizes and surface area that markedly limits diffusion. The cartilage calcifies with development of fissuring within its layers, and the end plate may separate from the vertebral body.[13,18,32,33] Impaired diffusion and transport leads to less absolute oxygen tension within the disk.[34] Although the metabolism of the disk is generally anaerobic, lactic acid production and accumulation increases with a tendency to a more acidic environment.[35,36] The accumulation of large degraded byproducts that exceed the diffusion capacity further obstructs any ability to clear wastes from the disk space and leads to diminished cellular metabolism and biosynthesis, resulting in impaired function. Thus, a vicious cycle is formed. Type II collagen within the end plate cartilage is diminished, whereas type X collagen, a phenotype associated with calcification, increases.[37]

The alterations within the nucleus initially are related to dehydration, with loss of cell viability caused by anaerobic metabolism and an increase in collagen fiber concentration.[14] As cell density decreases, less ECM is produced, water retention capacity is decreased, and dehydration occurs. PG content decreases, and formation of nonaggregated PG molecules increases. The ratio of chondroitin sulfate to keratan sulfate reverses with increased formation of the latter, which has less water-binding capacity.[38,39] An early adaptive increase in type II collagen production initially is found within the nucleus as well as in type I collagen fibers. Posttranslational modifications of collagen proteins also increase.

In the anulus, cell viability also eventually diminishes, with less ECM production and qualitative changes in collagen fibrils, although studies also suggest an early increase in type I collagen synthesis and PG messenger RNA (mRNA) and protein content that is interpreted as an initial but inadequate attempt at repair.[40-42] The ECM undergoes myxomatous degeneration with loss of normal organization of the collagen layers. The numbers of lamellae decrease, but the thickness of each layer and the spacing between the fiber bundles increase. Clefts form within the anulus near the edge of the disk and progress toward the nucleus.

Although the exact mechanism of pathogenesis is still under investigation, catabolic mediators often are produced spontaneously within the degenerating disk and include degradative enzymes such as matrix metalloproteinases (MMPs), oxygen free radicals, nitric oxide, interleukins, and prostaglandins.[14,18,43-48]

MMPs are a family of enzymes synthesized by connective tissue cells. They typically are regulated by a class of inhibitors known as tissue inhibitors of MMPs. It is hypothesized that as degenerative changes occur within the disk, the inhibitors become dysfunctional and allow the activity of MMPs.[49-52] The primary MMPs are stromelysin, more often found in the nucleus, and gelatinase and collagenase, found in the anulus.

Interleukins are a family of inflammatory cytokines that have been shown to decrease cellular metabolism and PG synthesis. High levels of IL-1, IL-6, and prostaglandin E$_2$ have been identified in herniated and degenerative disk tissue and may be capable of degradation by increasing the activity of other degradative enzymes.

Morphologic and Biomechanical Changes of Spondylosis

Kirkaldy-Willis and Farfan[53] described three clinical and biomechanical stages of spinal degeneration: initial early changes with mild dysfunction but no instability; later degenerative instability; and a final stabilization phase of osteophtye production and disk space collapse (Figure 5). Structural and biochemical changes have been correlated in several studies.[53,54]

The structural effects of loss of cell viability and ECM production are most evident on imaging studies, including loss of disk hydration on T2-weighted MRI, disk height loss and collapse, and instability. The earliest structural evidence of loss of water content within the nucleus is bulging of the anulus, and various radiographic degrees of changes have been described.[55] Compressive loads continue to be placed on the disk space as the nucleus desiccates and is no longer a self-contained hydrostatic structure. The nucleus becomes incapable of transferring load to the anulus, and the normal radial stress applied to the anulus is converted into axial stress.[56] The axial forces on the anulus lead to radial and circumferential tears within the overlapping lamellae. The height of the disk space diminishes as the extent of the degeneration and injury to the anulus increase. Annular bulging, which is often referred to as a contained herniated disk, into the spinal canal may develop. Disk height collapse leads to reduced stability from the outer anulus-vertebral body attachments, and increased motion may ensue. This additional mobility may stretch the disk further and intensify annular fraying and lamellar disorganization. End-plate thickening develops secondary to increased loads, bypassing the nucleus and along the periphery of the end plate where traction spurs or osteophytes may form.

The collapse of disk height also increases the load on the posterior facet joints, which undergo a degenerative process similar to appendicular synovium-lined joints. Cartilage surface erosion from altered mechanical pressure and motion leads to increased synovial fluid production and eventual osteophtye formation. Facet joint involvement in the absence of disk degeneration is unusual.

The combined ramifications of progressive disk degeneration and facet joint osteoarthritis include untoward static or dynamic translation of the vertebral bodies in the sagittal, axial, or coronal planes; severe disk height loss; or spinal stenosis of the central canal or foramina.[57-59] Fujiwara and associates[60] conducted a biomechanical and imaging study of human cadaver lumbar spinal motion segments and reported that axial

FIGURE 5

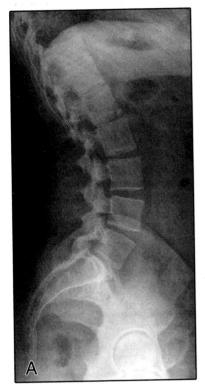 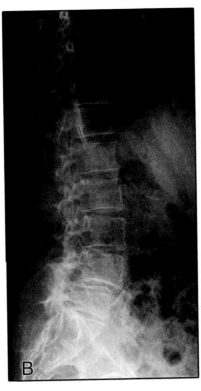 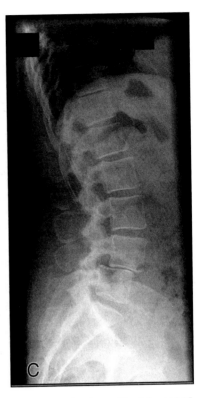

Lateral radiographs showing the degenerative stages defined by Kirkaldy-Willis and Farfan.[53] **A,** Early degenerative stage with minimal L4-L5 disk height loss and development of a "vacuum phenomenom." **B,** Instability stage with development of L4-L5 degenerative spondylolisthesis. **C,** End- stage degeneration with disk height collapse and stabilization.

rotation was most affected by disk degeneration and that segmental motion increased with the severity of degeneration but decreased at the extremes of disk degeneration.[61] Anterior translatory instability was shown to be related to disk and facet degeneration, whereas anteroposterior translatory instability or abnormal lateral tilting was more related to disk degeneration alone.[60,62]

CONCLUSIONS

The lumbar spine is an intricate, well-coordinated structure that provides pain-free motion and dissipates very high physiologic loads of the body. With extensive study, we now better understand both disk structure and composition at the cellular and molecular levels and their relationship with normal biomechanical func-

tion. The exact mechanisms of degeneration still are not known entirely, but a cascade of events is believed to be responsible for the age-related changes often seen. A basic understanding of normal lumbar anatomy and development and progression of spondylosis is important to a discussion of the clinical ramifications of diagnosis and treatment of common degenerative low back problems.

REFERENCES

1. White A, Panjabi M: *Clinical Biomechanics of the Spine,* ed 2. Philadelphia, PA, Lippincott, 1990.

2. Panjabi M, Goel V, Oxland T, et al: Human lumbar vertebrae: Quantitative three-dimensional anatomy. *Spine* 1992;17:299-306.

3. Berlemann U, Jeszenszky D, Buhler D, et al: Facet joint remodeling in degenerative spondylolisthesis: An investigation of joint orientation and tropism. *Eur Spine J* 1998;7:376-380.

4. Boden S, Martin C, Rudolph R, et al: Increase of motion between lumbar vertebrae after excision of the capsule and cartilage of the facets. *J Bone Joint Surg Am* 1994;76:1847-1853.

5. Adams M, Hutton W: The mechanical function of the lumbar apophyseal joints. *Spine* 1983;8:327-330.

6. Adams M, Hutton W, Scott J: The resistance to flexion of the lumbar intervertebral joint. *Spine* 1980;5:245-253.

7. Gunzberg R, Hutton W, Crane G, et al: Role of capsulo-ligamentous structures in rotation and combined flexion-rotation of the lumbar spine. *J Spinal Disord* 1992;5:1-7.

8. Panjabi M, Oxland T, Takata K, et al: Articular facets of the human spine. *Spine* 1993;18:1298-1310.

9. Hukins D, Kriby M, Sikoryn T, et al: Comparison of structure, mechanical properties, and functions of lumbar spinal ligaments. *Spine* 1990;15:787-795.

10. Lorenz M, Patwardhan A, Vanderby R: Load bearing characteristics of lumbar facets in normal and surgically altered spinal segments. *Spine* 1983;8:122-130.

11. Fujiwara A, Tamia K, Yoshida H, et al: Anatomy of the iliolumbar ligament. *Clin Orthop* 2000;380: 167-172.

12. Leong J, Luk K, Chow D, et al: The biomechanical functions of the iliolumbar ligament in maintaining stability of the lumbosacral junction. *Spine* 1987;12:669-674.

13. Bogduk N: *Clinical Anatomy of the Lumbar Spine and Sacrum: Moments of the Lumbar Spine.* Edinburgh, Scotland, Churchill Livingstone, 1997.

14. Guiot B, Fessler R: Molecular biology of degenerative disc disease. *Neurosurg* 2000;47:1034-1040.

15. Benjamin M, Ralphs J: Biology of fibrocartilage cells. *Int Rev Cytol* 2004;233:1-45.

16. Buckwalter J: Aging and degeneration of the human intervertebral disc. *Spine* 1995;20:1307-1314.

17. Holm S, Maroudas A, Urban J, Nachemson A: Nutrition of the intervertebral disc: Solute transport and metabolism. *Connect Tissue Res* 1981;8:101-109.

18. Katz M, Hargens A, Garfin S: Intervertebral disc nutrition: Diffusion versus convection. *Clin Orthop* 1986;210:243-245.

19. Chung S, Khan S, Diwan A: The molecular basis of intervertebral disc degeneration. *Orthop Clin North Am* 2003;34:209-219.

20. Boden S, Davis D, Dina T, et al: Abnormal magnetic resonance scans of the lumbar spine in asymptomatic patients: A prospective investigation. *J Bone Joint Surg Am* 1990;72:403-408.

21. Park J, Chang H, Kim K: Expression of fas ligand and apoptosis of disc cells in herniated lumbar disc tissue. *Spine* 2001;26:618-621.

22. Gruber H, Hanley E: Analysis of aging and degeneration of the human intervertebral disc: Comparison of surgical specimens with normal controls. *Spine* 1998;23:751-757.

23. Cassinelli E, Hall R, Kang J: Biochemistry of intervertebral disc degeneration and the potential for gene therapy application. *Spine J* 2001;1:205-214.

24. Freemont A, Watkins A, LeMaitre C, et al: Current understanding of cellular and molecular events in intervertebral disc degeneration: Implications for therapy. *J Pathol* 2002;196:374-379.

25. Adams M, Freeman B, Morrison H, et al: Mechanical initiation of intervertebral disc degeneration. *Spine* 2000;25:1625-1636.

26. Yu C, Tsai K, Hu W, et al: Geometric and morphological changes of the intervertebral disc under fatigue testing. *Clin Biomech* 2003;18:3-9.

27. Lotz J, Chin J: Intervertebral disc cell death is dependent on the magnitude and duration of spinal loading. *Spine* 2000;25:1477-1483.

28. Takao T, Iwaki T: A comparative study of localization of heat shock protein 27 and heat shock protein 72 in the developmental and degenerative intervertebral discs. *Spine* 2002;27:361-368.

29. Ariga K, Miyamoto S, Nakase T, et al: The relationship between apoptosis of endplate chondrocytes and aging and degeneration of the intervertebral disc. *Spine* 2001;26:2414-2420.

30. Kang J, Stefanovich-Racic M, McIntyre L, et al: Toward a biochemical understanding of human intervertebral disc degeneration and herniation: Contributions of nitric oxide, interleukins, prostaglandins E_2, and matrix metalloproteinases. *Spine* 1997;22:1065-1073.

31. Gruber H, Johnson T, Norton H, et al: The sand rat model for disc degeneration: Radiologic characterization of age-related changes. *Spine* 2002;27:230-234.

32. Horner H, Urban J: Effect of nutrient supply on the viability of cells from the nucleus pulposus of the intervertebral disc. *Spine* 2002;26:2543-2549.

33. Moore R: The vertebral end plate: What do we know? *Spine J* 2000;9:92-96.

34. Tanaka M, Nakahara S, Inoue H: A pathologic study of discs in the elderly: Separation between the cartilaginous end plate and the vertebral body. *Spine* 1993;11:1456-1462.

35. Roberts S, Urban J, Evans H, et al: Transport properties of the human cartilage endplate in relation to its composition and calcification. *Spine* 1996;21:415-420.

36. Bartels E, Fairbanks J, Winlove C, Urban J: Oxygen and lactate concentrations measured in vivo in the intervertebral disc. *Spine* 1998;23:1-7.

37. Boos N, Nerlich A, Wiest I, et al: Immunolocalization of type X collagen in human lumbar intervertebral discs during ageing and degeneration. *Histochem Cell Biol* 1997;108:471-480.

38. Hutton W, Elmer W, Boden S, Horton W, Carr K: Analysis of chondroitin sulfate in lumbar intervertebral discs at two different stages of degeneration as assessed by discogram. *J Spinal Disord* 1997;10:47-54.

39. Pearce RH, Grimmer BJ, Adams ME: Degeneration and the chemical composition of the human lumbar intervertebral disc. *J Orthop Res* 1987;5:198-205.

40. Ishihara H, Urban J: Effects of low oxygen concentrations and metabolic inhibitors on proteoglycan and protein synthesis. *J Orthop Res* 1999;17:829-835.

41. Gruber H, Hanley E: Ultrastructure of the human intervertebral disc during aging and degeneration: Comparison of surgical and control specimens. *Spine* 2002;27:798-805.

42. Cs-Szabo G, Ragasa-San Juan D, Turumella V, et al: Changes in mRNA and protein levels of proteoglycans of the annulus fibrosus and nucleus pulposus during intervertebral disc degeneration. *Spine* 2002;27:2212-2219.

43. Antoniou J, Steffen T, Nelson F, et al: The human lumbar intervertebral disc: Evidence for changes in the biosynthesis and denaturation of the extracellular matrix with growth, maturation, ageing, and degeneration. *J Clin Invest* 1996;98:996-1003.

44. Gruber H, Hanley E: Recent advances in disc cell biology. *Spine* 2003;28:186-193.

45. Casinelli E, Hall R, Kang J: Biochemistry of intervertebral disc degeneration and the potential for gene therapy applications. *Spine* 2001;26:205-214.

46. Kang J, Georgescu H, McIntyre-Larkin L, et al: Herniated cervical intervertebral discs spontaneously produce matrix metalloproteinases, nitric oxide, interleukin-6, and prostaglandin E$_2$. *Spine* 1995;20(suppl):2372-2378.

47. Liu G, Ishihara H, Osada R, et al: Nitric oxide mediates the change of proteoglycan synthesis in the human lumbar intervertebral disc in response to hydrostatic pressure. *Spine* 2001;26:134-141.

48. Matsui Y, Maeda M, Nakagami W, et al: The involvement of matrix metalloproteinases and inflammation in lumbar disc herniation. *Spine* 1998;23:863-869.

49. Roberts S, Caterson B, Meange J, et al: Matrix metalloproteinases and aggrecanase: Their role in disorders of the human intervertebral disc. *Spine* 2000;25:3005-3013.

50. Crean J, Roberts S, Jaffrey D, et al: Matrix metalloproteinases in the human intervertebral disc: Role in disc degeneration and scoliosis. *Spine* 1997;22:2877-2888.

51. Kanemoto M, Hukuda S, Komiya Y, et al: Immunohistochemical study of matrix metalloproteinase-3 and tissue inhibitor of metalloproteinase-1 in human intervertebral discs. *Spine* 1996;21:1-8.

52. Goupille P, Jayson M, Valat J, et al: Matrix metalloproteinases: The clue to intervertebral disc degeneration? *Spine* 1998;23:1612-1626.

53. Kirkaldy-Willis W, Farfan H: Instability of the lumbar spine. *Clin Orthop* 1982;165:110-123.

54. Boos N, Weissbach S, Rohrbach H, et al: Classification of age-related changes in lumbar intervertebral discs. *Spine* 2002;27:2631-2644.

55. Berlemann U, Gries N, Moore R: The relationship between height, shape and histologic changes in early disc degeneration of the lower lumbar discs. *Eur Spine J* 1998;7:212-217.

56. Umehara S, Tadano S, Abumi K, et al: Effects of degeneration on the elastic modulus distribution in the lumbar intervertebral disc. *Spine* 1996;21:811-819.

57. Pfirrmann C, Metzdorf A, Zanetti M, Holder J, Boos N: Magnetic resonance classification of lumbar intervertebral disc degeneration. *Spine* 2001;26:1873-1878.

58. Acaroglu E, Iatridis J, Setton L, et al: Degeneration and aging affect the tensile behavior of human lumbar annulus fibrosus. *Spine* 1995;20:2690-2701.

59. Mimura M, Panjabi M, Oxland T, et al: Disc degeneration affects the multidirectional flexibility of the lumbar spine. *Spine* 1994;19:1371-1380.

60. Fujiwara A, Lim T, An H, et al: The effect of disc degeneration and facet joint osteoarthritis on the segmental flexibility of the lumbar spine. *Spine* 2000;25:3036-3044.

61. Nachemson A, Schultz A, Berkson M: Mechanical properties of human lumbar spine motion segments: Influence of age, sex, disc level, and degeneration. *Spine* 1979;4:1-8.

62. Fujiwara A, Tamia K, An H, et al: The relationship of disc degeneration, facet joint osteoarthritis, and stability of the degenerative lumbar spine. *J Spinal Disord* 2000;13:444-450.

CHAPTER 2

EPIDEMIOLOGY, PATHOPHYSIOLOGY, AND CLINICAL EVALUATION OF LOW BACK PAIN

DAVID H. KIM, MD

TODD J. ALBERT, MD

ALAN S. HILIBRAND, MD

ALEXANDER R. VACCARO, MD

The study of low back pain (LBP) epidemiology and treatment is limited by a lack of consensus regarding the basic definition of terms and a prevalent misconception among researchers and practitioners that patients with LBP meaningfully can be thought of as a single group. LBP should be considered a symptom rather than a disorder. For the purposes of health care economics and policy, it has been helpful to combine all people with LBP into a single population to calculate aggregate figures such as time lost from work and societal costs. However, clinical studies reporting specific risk factors, sensitivity and specificity of diagnostic testing, or efficacy of treatment in which patients with LBP have been grouped together indiscriminately should be viewed with suspicion. LBP may be the dominant symptom of a variety of different medical conditions, including acute musculoligamentous strain, vertebral fracture, intervertebral disk injury or degeneration, spondylolysis, instability, or facet arthritis. The role of several of these conditions as pain generators remains highly controversial.

EPIDEMIOLOGY

Cross-sectional population studies provide consistent evidence of the extremely high prevalence of significant LBP in the general population. LBP is second only to headache as a frequent source of pain, with a reported lifetime prevalence of 60% to 80%, a 1-year prevalence of 56%, a 1-month prevalence of 19% to 43%, and a point prevalence of 15% to 30%.[1-9] The US Department of Health and Human Services estimates that chronic LBP limits the activity of nearly one third of the population to some degree at any given point in time.[8] Most LBP is described in terms of recurrent episodic pain that is mild to moderate in severity and of brief duration. This pattern has led to the suggestion that the fraction of painful days per year is a more informative concept than overall prevalence rates.[10]

Although varying prevalence rates are reported among different ethnic groups, much of the variation appears attributable to different definitions of LBP rather than to inherent differences among populations. A clear definition of LBP is required for accurate interpretation of any given study. LBP occurs posterior between the costal margin and the gluteal folds. Most studies of LBP focus on "nonspecific" LBP in which there is no well-defined pathology, and for inclusion of only clinically significant pain episodes, duration often is defined as a minimum of 24 hours.

Given similar definitions, most countries report comparable rates of LBP. The lifetime prevalence of LBP in England and Belgium is reported to be approximately 60%, whereas the rates in Scandinavia and Australia are somewhat higher, about 80%.[2,4,6,11-13] One-year prevalence rates in Tibet and Nigeria have been reported as 42% and 40%, respectively.[14,15]

A major limitation of retrospective studies is the potential for sampling and recall bias. Subpopulations selected for study are not necessarily representative of the population at large, and several factors have been identified as biasing recollection of previous pain episodes.[7,11,16-18] In particular, the current experience of LBP appears to enhance recall of previous episodes. Official government and industry figures also may be lower than self-reported population rates because many individuals do not seek medical treatment or file for disability benefits. A study from Denmark revealed that only 25% of individuals who reported having LBP sought medical attention, and fewer than 1 in 20 collected disability compensation.[19]

LBP is often viewed as a problem of middle-aged and older individuals, but recent epidemiologic studies suggest that the age of onset is distributed evenly between the second and fifth decades of life. Initial onset of significant LBP beyond the sixth decade is considered unusual.[7] LBP is a common finding among children, and by adolescence, its prevalence is similar to that found in adults. A prospective study of school-age children in Sweden revealed a 26% 1-year prevalence of back pain.[20] Burton and associates[21] conducted a prospective natural history study of LBP among adolescents and reported lifetime prevalence rates of 12% at age 11 years, increasing to 50% by age 15 years. Although the authors considered most adolescent LBP to be clinically insignificant, evidence is strong that the occurrence of significant LBP in childhood and adolescence predicts persistent recurrent pain in adulthood.[22]

Occupational Low Back Pain and Disability

LBP-related disability rates differ from LBP rates and vary from country to country and with time. Disability describes limitations in the performance of personal and job-related activities, and most experts believe that psychological, social, and political factors play a significant if not dominant role in determining a given individual's experience of disability.[23-26]

In the United States, LBP and lumbar spine disorders are the most common cause of lost time from work among individuals younger than age 45 years and the third most common among individuals between ages 45 and 65 years.[27] In Sweden, back pain is the most common cause of chronic illness among those younger than age 64 years and second only to vascular disease among those age 65 years and older.[7] In the United States, the 1-year prevalence of LBP disability is 7% to 14% of all workers. The National Health Interview Survey data[28] on more than 30,000 workers provides the best estimate of back pain-related time lost from work. In 1988, an estimated 17.6% of all workers (22.4 million people) were absent from work an aggregate 149 million days. Length of disability appears predictive of eventual return to work, with a 25% rate of return after 1 year of disability and negligible rates after 2 years.[29] At any given time, slightly more than 1% of the US population is considered permanently disabled as a result of LBP and another 1% is considered temporarily disabled.[30]

Large discrepancies in disability rates for different countries and over time have been attributed to distinct cultural attitudes toward pain and disability and varying policies regulating the distribution of disability benefits. Sweden reports significantly higher rates of back pain-related disability than the United States. In 1988, approximately 22.4 million Americans of working age lost an estimated 149 million days of work per year as a result of LBP for a rate of 6.7 days lost per worker per year.[28] By comparison, the 4.4 million working-age people in Sweden log about 50 million LBP-related sick days for a rate of 11.4 days per worker per year.[7,28] In England in 1992, the 1-year prevalence of LBP-related disability was reported as 11% for men and 7% for women, with a lifetime prevalence of 34% and 23%, respectively.[6] National disability data are affected strongly by changes in legislation. In Sweden, the official rate of work-related back injury fell by 80% between 1995 and 1996 in association with the introduction of stricter guidelines for identifying compensable LBP-related claims.[7]

LBP is considered the leading cause of time lost from work in industrialized countries.[31,32] In the United States alone, over a million workers' compensation claims for back pain are filed each year, a figure that represents nearly a third of the total number of claims. Total direct and indirect costs associated with LBP in the United States are estimated to exceed 100 billion dollars per year. Distribution of these costs is severely skewed, however, with 10% of individuals with chronic LBP responsible for more than 80% of the total costs.[33-35] The distribution of direct costs has been calculated for the period from 1988 to 1992 using an administrative database maintained by the National Council on Compensation Insurance.[36] This database also shows that health care costs are unevenly skewed, with the 20% of workers disabled for more than 4 months responsible for 60% of the direct costs. Diagnostic procedures were the highest single source of health care costs, responsible for 25% of those costs. Surgical treatment and physical therapy were second and third, responsible for 21% and 20% of costs, respectively.

Numerous prospective studies identify risk factors for transition to long-term disability and highlight psychological and socioeconomic characteristics of individuals.[37-43] Higher rates of recovery are associated with lower worker-reported stress levels and increased leisure-time exercise; cigarette smoking may be associated with poorer recovery rates.[44]

Fransen and associates[41] performed a prospective cohort study of 854 workers' compensation claimants in New Zealand to identify simple patient-reportable elements predictive of chronic back pain in a no-fault nonadversarial workers' compensation system.[41] Multiple independent determinants of chronicity were identified including the presence of severe leg pain (odds ratio [OR], 1.9), obesity (OR, 1.7), a job requiring lifting for at least 75% of the day (OR, 1.7), and lack of available light duty (OR, 1.7). The Oswestry disability index, a well-validated outcome measure for LBP, provided scores that were most highly predictive of chronicity (OR, 3.1 to 4). Similarly, a General Health Questionnaire-28 threshold score of 6, which is reported by the World Health Organization to be 80% sensitive and specific across cultures for the presence of

a significant psychological disorder, was found to be another independent risk factor of chronicity (OR, 1.9).[45]

Despite widespread opinion to the contrary, there is no strong epidemiologic evidence that the overall rate of LBP in the population has been increasing over time.[46] Review of the Scandinavian literature through 1954 revealed no significant increase in reported rates.[47] In the United States, LBP-related disability rates have fluctuated with no clear trend, although in one analysis of Washington state data, rates appear to have decreased by 30% in the 8 years from 1987 to 1995.[30]

Risk Factors

Hundreds of clinical studies have reported risk factors related to the development and persistence of nonspecific LBP. These studies focus primarily on patient-specific physical characteristics, physical activity, workplace environment, and psychological and socioeconomic status. Unfortunately, most studies are difficult or impossible to interpret because of significant shortcomings in methodology and inadequate statistical analysis. In many studies, the strongest predictor for the future occurrence of LBP appears to be the past experience of LBP, confirming the chronic episodic nature of most cases.[24,48-56]

Dozens of population studies strongly support an association between the repetitive performance of specific work-related tasks or postures and the development of LBP. Most studies implicate repetitive bending, lifting, or twisting maneuvers or sustained leaning or standing.[24,48,57-64] Pushing and pulling work tasks appear to be more strongly associated with shoulder pain than with LBP.[65,66] Truck driving, extensive car driving, and vibration exposure also may be risk factors.[67-69] Early studies suggesting that sitting while at work is a risk factor have been criticized for their cross-sectional design, and more recent studies suggest that sedentary work appears to have a neutral or possibly even protective effect against LBP.[17,70,71]

By definition, a cross-sectional survey assesses the status of an individual worker for the presence or absence of both exposure and disease at the same point in time. Because assessment of exposure and disease are made at a single point in time, time relationships and cause-effect relationships cannot be determined. At a minimum, extensive multiple regression analysis is required to eliminate spurious associations. An important source of bias in cross-sectional population studies is the "healthy worker" effect, described as either a susceptibility bias or selection bias in which healthy people tend to remain in their jobs, and those who change jobs generally tend to be less healthy.[17]

Hartvigsen and associates[17] conducted both cross-sectional and 5-year prospective cohort studies of 1,397 and 1,163 Danes, respectively, analyzing the proportion of workers who transferred between different workload groups. A very high job turnover rate was reported, with 67% of subjects making a significant change in their physical workload during the 5-year study period. Compared to workers with no LBP, a disproportionately high number of workers with LBP shifted from heavy physical work to sedentary work. Conversely, the group of workers shifting to heavy physical work from sedentary work during the same time period was disproportionately overrepresented by individuals without LBP. The result of this "healthy worker" effect was to inflate the ranks of sedentary workers with individuals who had LBP. A true strong association found between heavy physical work and LBP in the prospective arm of the study was eliminated in the cross-sectional study by movement of workers among labor groups, underscoring the inappropriateness of cross-sectional studies for the identification of occupational risk factors for LBP.

A principal goal of epidemiologic studies is to identify risk factors that may be amenable to intervention. Unfortunately, no evidence of a significant impact on rates of LBP has been reported in studies of ergonomic intervention in the workplace. One study followed the rates of LBP among nurses in two similar English hospitals and actually reported an increase in the prevalence of LBP in the hospital that pursued intensive ergonomic evaluation and major intervention.[72]

Sports and Recreational Activities

Evidence that regular exercise and higher levels of physical fitness reduce the lifetime risk of developing LBP is limited.[73-81] Conflicting data on the relationship between regular running and walking and LBP have been reported.[76,82,83] The prevalence of radiographic disk degeneration is higher in athletes than in nonathletes, and the rate of symptomatic spondylolysis is particularly pronounced in individuals who participate in certain sports such as gymnastics and weightlifting.[84] In a longitudinal study of an industrial worker population, Stevenson and associates[85] reported that maintaining a high level of physical fitness had a significant effect on reducing rates of first-time LBP.

Obesity

Overall, the evidence that obesity is a risk factor for LBP is weak, with many studies failing to identify a significant association.[69,86-90] A systematic review of 65 studies revealed that 32% reported a statistically significant but weak positive association.[90] A cross-sectional survey from the Netherlands of 12,905 subjects found an association between obesity and LBP in women but not in men.[91] Deyo and Bass,[92] using national survey data and multiple regression analysis, identified obesity as an independent risk factor with an odds ratio of 1.7 for individuals considered the most obese 20%. No acceptable study reported an odds ratio greater than 2, and after applying Bradford Hill's criteria for causality (strength of association, dose-response relationship, temporality, reversibility, and consistency), the authors concluded that a causal relationship could not be established by the available literature.

Nevertheless, there is stronger evidence that obesity contributes to pain chronicity once an episode of LBP has begun. Leboeuf-Yde and associates,[89] in a study using data from the Danish Twin Register of 29,424 twin subjects, reported a consistent but weak positive association between obesity and LBP, with a stronger association for the risk of developing LBP lasting more than 30 days. However, no significant difference in risk was identified in monozygotic twins who were dissimilar in weight. The authors concluded that obesity was modestly associated with chronic or recurrent pain but that the monozygotic twin data indicated a causal relationship was unlikely.

Cigarette Smoking

Despite a good biologic animal model of degenerative disk disease based on nicotine administration and multiple plausible biologic mechanisms, epidemiologic evidence that cigarette smoking is a significant risk factor for LBP remains inconclusive. Proposed but unproved mechanisms linking the two include increased intradiskal pressure from coughing, reduction in vertebral blood flow, impaired fibrinolysis, and decreased bone mineralization resulting in microfracture.[93] Most studies that report cigarette smoking as a significant risk factor are cross-sectional in design.[24,54,88,93-102] Using national survey data and multiple regression analysis, Deyo and Bass[92] identified cigarette smoking as an independent risk factor. The risk increased with duration of smoking and was particularly pronounced in individuals younger than age 45 years. Ten years after smoking cessation, LBP rates in these individuals equalized with those of nonsmokers. Leboeuf-Yde and associates[103] conducted a questionnaire study of more than 25,000 twin subjects enrolled in the Danish Twin Register and reported a significant positive association between smoking and LBP that appeared stronger with longer durations of LBP. However, no significant difference was found in monozygotic twin pairs who were discordant with respect to smoking status, and smoking cessation was not associated with a decreased prevalence of LBP. The authors concluded that the association was spurious, and a causal relationship could not be supported.

Psychosocial Factors

Many studies identify psychosocial factors such as emotional stress as risk factors for LBP.[58,104] Job dissatisfaction, in particular, has been repeatedly associated with work-related LBP and disability.[50,51,60,62,79,105-110] A cross-sectional study of 5,781 members of the 1958 British birth cohort identified psychological distress at age 23 years as the single strongest risk factor for LBP at ages 32 to 33 years.[94] Another prospective study of 114 nurses in their first year of practice included a subset of 24 nurses whose urinary catecholamine levels were measured at regular intervals. Low control at work and increased activation of the sympathetic-adrenal medullary system as measured by urinary catecholamine level was associated with increased risk for LBP.[111]

Numerous studies suggest that low educational status may be related to LBP, but this association remains controversial. A review by Dionne and associates[112] of 64 studies specifically addressing the relationship between level of formal education and LBP concluded that the available evidence supports an association between low education and increased risk for disabling LBP. There appears to be a stronger association with duration of symptoms and recurrence of LBP than for onset of LBP. Various mechanisms have been proposed to explain this finding, including covariation with other behavioral and environmental risk factors, differences in types of occupation, and more limited access to health care.

Psychological Factors

Psychological and mood disorders such as anxiety and depression also have been associated with LBP.[113] The biopsychosocial model of nonspecific LBP has been espoused by a number of practitioners and prioritizes nonphysical characteristics as determinants of LBP behavior, chronicity, and treatment outcome.[114,115] Pincus and associates[116] produced the most comprehensive and critical review of the role of psychological factors in the development of chronic LBP. Only six studies met rigorous criteria for methodology and analysis. The most consistent finding among these studies was that psychological distress, symptoms of depression, and depressive mood were significantly predictive of poor outcome independent of pain and function at baseline. Somatization was found to be predictive in two studies. Calculation of Cohen's effect-size statistic revealed a moderate effect size for psychological distress and depressive mood and a variable effect size for somatization.[116]

Pregnancy

LBP is a common complaint during pregnancy and affects an estimated 68% of pregnant women.[117] Although typically mild to moderate in severity and generally considered to have a favorable long-term prognosis, the rate of persistent pain at 2 years after delivery may be as high as 21%.[118] Risk factors that have been associated with LBP during pregnancy include younger age and previous history of LBP with or without pregnancy.[117] Persistent pain after delivery has been associated with older age and higher weight.[118]

LBP in Childhood

Proposed risk factors for LBP in childhood are similar to those in adults and include heavy lifting, repetitive or sustained bending, sustained sitting, and cigarette smoking.[119] An association between childhood back pain and parental back pain also has been reported.[120] A prospective cohort study of 1,046 British schoolchildren aged 11 to 14 years sought to identify risk factors for new onset of LBP at 1-year follow-up.[121] Significant risk factors included psychosocial difficulty or conduct problems at baseline as well as high numbers of somatic symptoms at baseline (ie, abdominal pain, headache, and sore throat). Schoolbag weight was not reported to be strongly associated. Although studies have suggested between 30% and 54% of elementary school children carry backpacks in excess of 15% of their body weight, and parents frequently express concern about their children carrying heavy backpacks to school, the available clinical evidence from multiple studies is weak.[119,121-124]

Sciatica

The presence of associated sciatica in patients with LBP is critically important in determining diagnosis, treatment, and prognosis. Unfortunately, most population studies of LBP fail to adequately distinguish true sciatica, defined as pain distribution down the lower extremity in a radicular pattern, from the more common nonspecific referred pain. Lifetime prevalence rates for leg pain associated with back pain have been variably reported between 14% and 40%, but these figures are likely inflated by a high percentage of individuals with referred pain. Heliovaara and associates[125] from Finland applied strict criteria for identifying episodes of true sciatica and reported in men a 77% lifetime prevalence of back pain, a 35% rate of associated lower extremity pain, and a 5% rate of true sciatica. In women, the figures were 74%, 45%, and 4%, respectively.

Although sciatica traditionally has been regarded as having a generally favorable long-term prognosis, recent studies suggest a surprisingly high rate of chronicity. In a prospective cohort study of 622 French electrical and gas workers reporting sciatica, 53% reported persistent symptoms after 4 years.[126] Driving in excess of 2 hours per day, carrying heavy loads, history of psychosomatic illness, and a history of sciatica for at least 1 year all predicted worse outcome.

Risk Factors for Sciatica

Few epidemiologic studies focus on the risk factors for onset and persistence of sciatica as opposed to LBP. Miranda and associates[82] reported a 1-year prospective cohort study comparing 2,077 workers free of sciatica to 327 workers with sciatica. Significant risk factors for sciatica onset included advanced age, cigarette smoking, work-related trunk torsion, active walking as a component of regular physical exercise, and self-reported "mental stress." Risk factors for persistent sciatica included

age, history of smoking, active jogging, mental stress, and job dissatisfaction. In general, the authors believed that the characteristics of physical work were more significant risk factors for the onset of sciatica, whereas psychosocial factors were more important in terms of its persistence.

Natural History

As previously described, LBP becomes a relatively common complaint during early adolescence and appears to maintain a steady incidence of new onset episodes through middle age. European studies report a prevalence of 10%, increasing to 13% through adolescence.[119,127] The prevalence of LBP in adulthood is so high that it should be considered a part of normal life experience in most individuals. Although many patients recall a specific event such as a lifting or twisting maneuver temporally related to the acute onset of pain, many do not report any history of antecedent trauma.

Because nonspecific LBP is not a clearly defined pathologic entity, natural history studies are difficult to interpret. Even with the use of advanced imaging techniques such as MRI, the exact pathologic basis for pain in most patients cannot be clearly established.[128] Without an established diagnosis, treatment remains nonspecific and symptomatic in nature. Fortunately, most LBP is relatively benign and characterized by mild to moderate pain that is readily controlled by a combination of brief periods of rest, activity modification, occasional application of modalities such as heat therapy, and nonnarcotic pain medication.[129] Of patients with LBP, 42% experience persistent pain on an annual basis.[130] Although nonspecific LBP tends to recur episodically for many years, the overall prognosis for recovery from any given episode is considered good, and long-term outcome appears similar, regardless of treatment.

The natural history of LBP-related disability is distinct from that of LBP alone. Specific work activity and workplace elements play a role, and psychosocial factors have been shown to be significant determinants of chronicity. Chronic LBP is associated with significantly greater disability that often increases with time.[130-133]

The natural history of spondylolysis and spondylolisthesis has been reported in a 45-year longitudinal study of 500 first-grade children unselected for any kind of LBP.[134] Over the course of the follow-up period, 30 subjects (6%) were diagnosed with spondylolysis. No significant difference was identified in SF-36 scores between subjects with spondylolysis and spondylolisthesis and the general age-matched population. The rate of slip progression in patients with spondylolisthesis steadily declined with each passing decade, and there was no association between slip progression and LBP, although no subject experienced slippage beyond 40%. Nonsurgical treatment appears adequate to control symptoms in approximately 60% of patients with spondylolisthesis and LBP.[135]

PATHOPHYSIOLOGY

Spondylosis and Degenerative Disk Disease

Spondylosis and disk degeneration are characteristic findings on plain radiographs, CT, and MRI in most patients with nonspecific LBP. Spondylosis refers to age-related structural degeneration of the spinal column. Specific elements that often are apparent on radiographs include marginal vertebral body osteophytes, facet-joint hypertrophy, ligamentum flavum hypertrophy, and multidirectional spondylolisthesis. Implicit in the concept of spondylosis is the idea that these anatomic changes reflect the accumulated experience of biomechanical stresses over the course of an individual's lifetime.

Degenerative disk disease currently is one of the most controversial topics in spinal medicine, with little consensus in terms of definition, evaluation, diagnosis, or treatment. It is well established that histologic and radiographic changes in the lumbar intervertebral disk are common enough in asymptomatic individuals that such changes should be considered a normal part of the aging process. The prevalence of specific changes, including disk desiccation, protrusion, loss of height, and fissuring, appears to increase with age and does not necessarily reflect the presence or progression of symptomatic LBP.[136-138] Boden and associates[139] evaluated MRI scans of 67 subjects without back pain and identified disk degeneration or bulging in 35% of asymptomatic 20- to 39-year old individuals, with progressively higher rates in older age groups. MRI findings of extruded disk material, nerve root compression, or moderate to severe stenosis are more likely to corre-

late with specific symptoms and objective clinical findings.

Annular ruptures or tears as an anatomic correlate for LBP have been a target of considerable controversy. Many studies report an association between the presence of an annular tear and clinically significant LBP.[140,141] Histologic studies have identified nerve ingrowth in association with annular tears, suggesting an anatomic basis for discogenic LBP.[142] Moneta and associates[143] reviewed the results of 833 diskograms in 306 candidates for lumbar spinal surgery and reported an association between tears of the outer anulus fibrosus and similar or exact pain reproduction. Although CT diskography is considered the gold standard for identification of an annular tear, a "high intensity zone" (HIZ) in the outer anulus appears to be the correlative MRI finding.[144] The sensitivity, specificity, positive predictive value, and negative predictive value of the HIZ lesion on MRI for a concordantly painful posterior annular tear have been estimated at 27%, 95%, 89%, and 47%, respectively.[144] Videman and associates[141] performed a retrospective MRI study of 115 monozygotic twins evaluating several parameters, including disk height, bulging, herniations, annular tears, osteophytes, stenosis, and end-plate changes, and reported that diminished disk height and annular tears were the only significant parameters predicting LBP.

Transitional Lumbosacral Anatomy

Transitional lumbosacral anatomy, also known as Bertolotti's syndrome, is present in 12% to 21% of the population.[145-149] Typically, the fifth lumbar segment is partially or entirely sacralized or the first sacral segment is partially lumbarized with a persistent caudal disk space. Increased regional stress at the segment proximal to the transitional segment has been suggested as a potential risk factor for development of disk disorders and back pain. In the presence of a transitional, partially sacralized L5 vertebra, a high intercrestal line and a long L5 transverse process have been associated with an increased prevalence of radiographic L4-5 disk degeneration.[150] Multiple studies have suggested an increased risk of disk herniation at the proximal level and a possible protective effect with reduced rates of degeneration at the caudal level.[145,146,151,152] Cross-sectional studies, however, have failed to identify an association between transitional vertebrae and LBP.[153]

Clinical Evaluation

Given the benign nature and favorable long-term prognosis of most episodes of LBP, advanced imaging studies and intervention beyond symptomatic management should be deferred for at least 4 to 6 weeks in almost all affected individuals. Early plain radiographs should be considered if significant trauma is involved, and early MRI may be appropriate in patients with a history of cancer, recent infection, or systemic symptoms or signs of illness such as fever, chills, or unintentional weight loss. Significant or progressive neurologic deficit on examination also is an indication for early advanced imaging studies.

Clinical evaluation of the patient begins with general observation of mood, affect, and behavior. Waddell and associates[154] repopularized the use of nonorganic signs, ie, examination findings suggesting a nonorganic component to a patient's back pain. They originally described five clinically useful signs: tenderness, simulation, distraction, regional disturbances, and overreaction. The presence of three out of five signs suggests a strong nonorganic contribution and the possible need for supplemental psychological evaluation.

Nonspecific LBP is a diagnosis of exclusion, and therefore, the patient history and physical examination should be designed to determine the likelihood that a more specific clinicopathologic process is present. The location, quality, severity, and duration of pain are fundamental diagnostic elements. Radiation of pain below the level of the knee, especially in a radicular pattern, is highly suggestive of sciatica and the potential for anatomic nerve root compression by a disk herniation. Lower extremity pain that remains above the knee is more often referred pain from degenerative disk disease or spondylotic arthropathy. Aggravating and alleviating factors are diagnostically relevant. Chronic or episodic lumbar pain exacerbated by leaning forward may indicate degenerative disk disease. Valsalva maneuvers such as coughing or sneezing increase intradiskal pressure and often provoke pain from a discogenic source. Back pain that is exacerbated by neutral posture or lumbar extension may be originating from spondylolysis, facet degeneration, or spinal stenosis. The possibility of tumor or infection must always be considered and carefully assessed. A previous history of LBP complaints, including duration and response to treatments, is often predictive for eventual course of the current LBP episode.

The social history is a crucial component of the evaluation of LBP. Employment status, job satisfaction, and the presence of potential secondary gain issues such as history of a motor vehicle accident or active litigation must tactfully be elicited. The physical examination should include height, weight, and general body habitus. Alignment and gait should be assessed. Skin, particularly over the lumbosacral area, should be inspected for congenital lesions. Firm palpation of the lumbar region often elicits nonspecific tenderness over the paraspinal musculature or posterior superior iliac spines. Distinct midline tenderness over the spinous process suggests the possibility of a fracture or other osseous lesion. Reports of significant pain with light touch or light pinching of the skin is considered a positive Waddell's sign, carrying the potential for nonorganic illness. Thoracolumbar range of motion should be recorded, but limited motion is not particularly diagnostic.

A straight leg raise test should be performed with the patient in the seated and supine positions. Elicitation of pain while the patient is supine but not while he or she is seated, particularly while the examiner appears to be focused on another aspect of the examination, is another Waddell's sign. In young patients, a positive straight leg test is both sensitive and specific for disk herniation, but this may not be the case in patients older than age 50 years.

Finally, a thorough neurologic examination should be performed. Radicular weakness and/or dermatomal sensory loss suggest a possible disk herniation, whereas regional, nondermatomal sensory loss, or whole extremity weakness is considered another positive Waddell's sign.

Summary

Nonspecific LBP represents an enormous problem in terms of public health and socioeconomic costs. The lifetime prevalence of significant LBP is between 60% and 80% and has remained relatively constant across cultures and times. The tremendous number of clinical studies published provides confusing and often conflicting information regarding specific risk factors, and individual reports should be viewed carefully. Meta-analyses typically discard 45% to 95% of published studies as unacceptable for aggregate analysis because of significant methodologic or statistical flaws. In particular, cross-sectional studies of specific worker populations should be interpreted with caution because of the "healthy worker" effect. Reasonably good evidence implicates heavy manual labor with repetitive bending, lifting, and twisting as a risk factor for development of nonspecific LBP. The evidence for cigarette smoking and obesity as significant risk factors is relatively weaker. Once LBP is present, the duration of symptoms appears significantly affected by various psychosocial factors such as depression and job satisfaction.

Meaningful epidemiologic analysis of LBP is severely challenged by the lack of clearly defined and meaningful clinicopathologic terms. The utility of specific diagnostic tests such as MRI and diskography and the efficacy of specific interventions from physical therapy to surgery cannot be assessed adequately until understanding of the condition eliminates use of the term "nonspecific LBP."

REFERENCES

1. Cassidy JD, Carroll LJ, Cote P: The Saskatchewan Health and Back Pain Survey: The prevalence of low back pain and related disability in Saskatchewan adults. *Spine* 1998;23:1860-1867.

2. Papageorgiou AC, Croft PR, Ferry S, Jayson MI, Silman AJ: Estimating the prevalence of low back pain in the general population: Evidence from the South Manchester Back Pain Survey. *Spine* 1995;20:1889-1894.

3. Shekelle PG, Markovich M, Louie R: An epidemiologic study of episodes of back pain care. *Spine* 1995;20:1668-1673.

4. Skovron ML, et al: Sociocultural factors and back pain. *Spine* 1995;19:129-137.

5. Von Korff M, et al: An epidemiologic comparison of pain complaints. *Pain* 1988;32:173-183.

6. Walsh K, Cruddas M, Coggon D: Low back pain in eight areas of Britain. *J Epidemiol Community Health* 1992;46:227-230.

7. Nachemson A: Epidemiology and the economics of low back pain, in Herkowitz HN, et al, (eds): *The Lumbar Spine*. Philadelphia, PA, Lippincott Williams & Wilkins, 2004, pp 3-10.

8. Healthy People 2010 [database]. Washington, DC, US Department of Health and Human Services, 2003.

9. Taylor H, Curran NM: *The Nuprin Pain Report*. New York, NY, Louis Harris and Associates, 1985, pp 1-233.

10. Croft PR, et al: Psychological distress and low back pain: Evidence from a prospective study in the general population. *Spine* 1995;20:2731-2737.

11. Biering-Sorensen F, Hilden J: Reproducibility of the history of low back trouble. *Spine* 1984;9:280-286.

12. Bergenudd H, Nilsson B: Back pain in middle age; occupational workload and psychologic factors: An epidemiologic survey. *Spine* 1988;13:58-60.

13. Walker BF, Muller R, Grant WD: Low back pain in Australian adults: Health provider utilization and care seeking. *J Manipulative Physiol Ther* 2004;27:327-335.

14. Hoy D, et al: Low back pain in rural Tibet. *Lancet* 2003;361:225-226.

15. Omokhodion FO: Low back pain in a rural community in South West Nigeria. *West Afr J Med* 2002;21:87-90.

16. Haas M, Nyiendo J, Aickin M: One-year trend in pain and disability relief recall in acute and chronic ambulatory low back pain patients. *Pain* 2002;95:83-91.

17. Hartvigsen J, et al: The association between physical workload and low back pain clouded by the "healthy worker" effect. *Spine* 2001;26:1788-1793.

18. Seferlis T, et al: Acute low-back pain patients exhibit a fourfold increase in sick leave for other disorders: A case-control study. *J Spinal Disord* 1999;12:280-286.

19. Lonnberg F: The management of back problems among the population. II: Therapists' and patients' perception of the disease. *Ugeskr Laeger* 1997;159:215-221.

20. Brattberg G: Back pain and headache in Swedish schoolchildren: A longitudinal study. *Pain Clin* 1993;6:157-162.

21. Burton KA, et al: The natural history of low back pain in adolescents. *Spine* 1996;21:2323-2328.

22. Harreby M, et al: Are radiologic changes in the thoracic and lumbar spine of adolescents risk factors for low back pain in adults? A 25-year prospective cohort study of 640 school children. *Spine* 1995;20:2298-2302.

23. Waddell G, Aylward M, Sawney P: *Back Pain, Incapacity of Work and Social Security Benefits: An International Literature Review and Analysis.* London, Royal Society of Medicine Press, 2002.

24. Tubach F, et al: Risk factors for sick leave due to low back pain: A prospective study. *J Occup Environ Med* 2002;44:451-458.

25. Magora A: An investigation of the relation between low back pain and occupation: III. Physical requirements: Sitting, standing, and weight lifting. *Ind Med* 1972;41:5-9.

26. Magora A: Investigation of the relation between low back pain and occupation: V. Psychological aspects. *Scand J Rehabil Med* 1973;5:191-196.

27. Kelsey JL, White AA III: Epidemiology and impact of low-back pain. *Spine* 1980;5:133-142.

28. Guo HR, Tanaka S, Cameron LL, et al: Back pain among workers in the United States: National estimates and workers at high risk. *Am J Industr Med* 1995;28:591-602.

29. McGill CM: Industrial back problems: A control program. *J Occup Med* 1968;10:174-178.

30. Murphy PL, Volinn E: Is occupational low back pain on the rise? *Spine* 1999;24:691-697.

31. Battie MC, Bigos SJ: Industrial back pain complaints: A broader perspective. *Orthop Clin North Am* 1991;22: 273-282.

32. Guo HR, et al: Back pain prevalence in US industry and estimates of lost workdays. *Am J Public Health* 1999;89:1029-1035.

33. Hashemi L, et al: Length of disability and cost of workers' compensation low back pain claims. *J Occup Environ Med* 1997;39:937-945.

34. Murphy PL, Courtney TK: Low back pain disability: Relative costs by antecedent and industry group. *Am J Ind Med* 2000;37:558-571.

35. Volinn E, Van Koevering D, Loeser JD: Back sprain in industry: The role of socioeconomic factors in chronicity. *Spine* 1991;16:542-548.

36. Williams DA, et al: Health care and indemnity costs across the natural history of disability in occupational low back pain. *Spine* 1998;23:2329-2336.

37. Cats-Baril WL, Frymoyer JW: Identifying patients at risk of becoming disabled because of low-back pain: The Vermont Rehabilitation Engineering Center predictive model. *Spine* 1991;16:605-607.

38. Coste J, et al: Clinical course and prognostic factors in acute low back pain: An inception cohort study in primary care practice. *BMJ* 1994;308:577-580.

39. Gallagher RM, et al: Determinants of return-to-work among low back pain patients. *Pain* 1989;39:55-67.

40. Gatchel RJ, Polatin PB, Mayer TG: The dominant role of psychosocial risk factors in the development of chronic low back pain disability. *Spine* 1995;20:2702-2709.

41. Fransen M, et al: Risk factors associated with the transition from acute to chronic occupational back pain. *Spine* 2002;27:92-98.

42. Lehmann TR, Spratt KF, Lehmann KK: Predicting long-term disability in low back injured workers presenting to a spine consultant. *Spine* 1993;18:1103-1112.

43. van der Weide WE, et al: Prognostic factors for chronic disability from acute low-back pain in occupational health care. *Scand J Work Environ Health* 1999;25:50-56.

44. Oleske DM, et al: Factors affecting recovery from work-related, low back disorders in autoworkers. *Arch Phys Med Rehabil* 2004;85:1362-1364.

45. Goldberg DP, et al: The validity of two versions of the GHQ in the WHO study of mental illness in general health care. *Psychol Med* 1997;27:191-197.

46. Allan DB, Waddell G: An historical perspective on low back pain and disability. *Acta Orthop Scand* 1989;234(suppl):1-23.

47. Leboeuf-Yde C, Lauritsen JM: The prevalence of low back pain in the literature: A structured review of 26 Nordic studies from 1954 to 1993. *Spine* 1995;20:2112-2118.

48. Hellsing AL, Bryngelsson IL: Predictors of musculoskeletal pain in men: A twenty-year follow-up from examination at enlistment. *Spine* 2000;25:3080-3086.

49. Bigos SJ, et al: A longitudinal, prospective study of industrial back injury reporting. *Clin Orthop* 1992;279:21-34.

50. Bigos SJ, et al: A prospective study of work perceptions and psychosocial factors affecting the report of back injury. *Spine* 1991;16:1-6.

51. Burdorf A, Sorock G: Positive and negative evidence of risk factors for back disorders. *Scand J Work Environ Health* 1997;23:243-256.

52. Frank JW, et al: Disability resulting from occupation low back pain: Part I. What do we know about primary prevention? A review of the scientific evidence on prevention before disability begins. *Spine* 1996;21:2908-2917.

53. Frank JW, et al: Disability resulting from occupational low back pain: Part II. What do we know about secondary prevention? A review of the scientific evidence on prevention after disability begins. *Spine* 1996;21:2918-2929.

54. Frymoyer JW, Pope MH, Clements JH: Risk factors in low back pain: An epidemiologic review. *J Bone Joint Surg Am* 1983;65:213-218.

55. Mannion AF, Dolan P, Adams MA: Psychological questionnaires: Do "abnormal" scores precede or follow first-time low back pain. *Spine* 1996;21:2603-2611.

56. Troup JDG, Martin JW, Lloyd CEF: Back pain in industry: A prospective survey. *Spine* 1981;6:61-69.

57. Lu JL: Risk factors for low back pain among Filipino manufacturing workers and their anthropometric measurements. *Appl Occup Environ Hyg* 2003;18:170-176.

58. Yip YB, Ho SC, Chan SG: Identifying risk factors for low back pain (LBP) in Chinese middle-aged women: A case-control study. *Health Care Women Int* 2004;25:358-369.

59. Damkot DK, et al: The relationship between work history, work environment and low-back pain in men. *Spine* 1984;9:395-399.

60. Latza U, Pfahlberg A, Gefeller O: Impact of repetitive manual materials handling and psychosocial work factors on the future prevalence of chronic low-back pain among construction workers. *Scand J Work Environ Health* 2002;28:314-323.

61. Sobti A, et al: Occupational physical activity and long-term risk of musculoskeletal symptoms: A national survey of post office pensioners. *Am J Ind Med* 1997;32:76-83.

62. Hoogendoorn WE, et al: High physical work load and low job satisfaction increase the risk of sickness absence due to

low back pain: Results of a prospective cohort study. *Occup Environ Med* 2002;59:323-328.

63. Lee P, et al: Low back pain: Prevalence and risk factors in an industrial setting. *J Rheumatol* 2001;28:346-351.

64. Lotters F, et al: Model for the work-relatedness of low-back pain. *Scand J Work Environ Health* 2003;29:431-440.

65. Hoozemans MJ, et al: Pushing and pulling in association with low back and shoulder complaints. *Occup Environ Med* 2002;59:696-702.

66. Hoozemans MJ, et al: Low-back and shoulder complaints among workers with pushing and pulling tasks. *Scand J Work Environ Health* 2002;28:293-303.

67. Kelsey JL, Hardy RJ: Driving of motor vehicles as a risk factor for acute herniated lumbar intervertebral disc. *Am J Epidemiol* 1975;102:63-73.

68. Matsui H, et al: Risk indicators of low back pain among workers in Japan: Association of familial and physical factors with low back pain. *Spine* 1997;22:1242-1248.

69. Bovenzi M, Zadini A: Self-reported low back symptoms in urban bus drivers exposed to whole-body vibration. *Spine* 1992;17:1048-1059.

70. Hartvigsen J, et al: Is sitting-while-at-work associated with low back pain? A systematic, critical literature review. *Scand J Public Health* 2000;28:230-239.

71. Hoogendoorn WE, et al: Physical load during work and leisure time as risk factors for back pain. *Scand J Work Environ Health* 1999;25:385-386.

72. Smedley J, et al: Risk factors for incident neck and shoulder pain in hospital nurses. *Occup Environ Med* 2003;60:864-869.

73. Harreby M, et al: Low back pain and physical exercise in leisure time in 38-year-old men and women: A 25-year prospective cohort study of 640 school children. *Eur Spine J* 1997;6:181-186.

74. Kool J, et al: Exercise reduces sick leave in patients with non-acute non-specific low back pain: A meta-analysis. *J Rehabil Med* 2004;36:49-62.

75. Picavet HS, Schuit AJ: Physical inactivity: A risk factor for low back pain in the general population? *J Epidemiol Community Health* 2003;57:517-518.

76. Lahad A, et al: The effectiveness of four interventions for the prevention of low back pain. *JAMA* 1994;272:1286-1291.

77. Cady LD, et al: Strength and fitness and subsequent back injuries in firefighters. *J Occup Med* 1979;21:269-272.

78. Leino PI: Does leisure time physical activity prevent low back disorders? A prospective study of metal industry employees. *Spine* 1993;18:863-871.

79. McQuade KJ, Turner JA, Buchner DM: Physical fitness and chronic low back pain: An analysis of the relationships among fitness, functional limitations, and depression. *Clin Orthop* 1988;233:198-204.

80. Mostardi RA, et al: Isokinetic lifting strength and occupational injury: A prospective study. *Spine* 1992;17:189-193.

81. Battie MC, et al: Isometric lifting strength as a predictor of industrial back pain reports. *Spine* 1989;14:851-856.

82. Miranda H, et al: Individual factors, occupational loading, and physical exercise as predictors of sciatic pain. *Spine* 2002;27:1102-1109.

83. Woolf SK, et al: The Cooper River Bridge Run Study of low back pain in runners and walkers. *J South Orthop Assoc* 2002;11:136-143.

84. Bono CM: Low-back pain in athletes. *J Bone Joint Surg Am* 2004;86:382-396.

85. Stevenson JM, et al: A longitudinal study of the development of low back pain in an industrial population. *Spine* 2001;26:1370-1377.

86. Biering-Sorensen F: Physical measurements as risk indicators for low-back trouble over a one-year period. *Spine* 1984;9:106-119.

87. Smedley J, et al: Prospective cohort study of predictors of incident low back pain in nurses. *BMJ* 1997;314:1225-1228.

88. Heliovaara M, et al: Determinants of sciatica and low-back pain. *Spine* 1991;16:608-614.

89. Leboeuf-Yde C, Kyvik KO, Bruun NH: Low back pain and lifestyle: Part II. Obesity: Information from a population-based sample of 29,424 twin subjects. *Spine* 1999;24:779-784.

90. Leboeuf-Yde C: Body weight and low back pain: A systematic literature review of 56 journal articles reporting on 65 epidemiologic studies. *Spine* 2000;25:226-237.

91. Han TS, et al: The prevalence of low back pain and associations with body fatness, fat distribution and height. *Int J Obes Relat Metab Disord* 1997;21:600-607.

92. Deyo RA, Bass JE: Lifestyle and low-back pain: The influence of smoking and obesity. *Spine* 1989;14:501-506.

93. Goldberg MS, Scott SC, Mayo NE: A review of the association between cigarette smoking and the development of nonspecific back pain and related outcomes. *Spine* 2000;25:995-1014.

94. Power C, et al: Predictors of low back pain onset in a prospective British study. *Am J Public Health* 2001;91:1671-1678.

95. Biering-Sorensen F, Thomsen C: Medical, social and occupational history, risk indicators for low-back trouble in a general population. *Spine* 1986;11:720-725.

96. Ferguson SA, Marras WS: A literature review of low back disorder surveillance measures and risk factors. *Clin Biomech* 1997;12:211-216.

97. Leboeuf-Yde C: Smoking and low back pain. *Spine* 1999;24:1463-1470.

98. Andersson H, Ejlertsson G, Leden I: Widespread musculoskeletal chronic pain associated with smoking: An

epidemiological study in a general rural population. *Scand J Rehabil Med* 1998;30:185-191.

99. Scott SC, et al: The association between cigarette smoking and back pain in adults. *Spine* 1999;24:1090-1098.

100. Boshuizen HC, et al: Do smokers get more back pain? *Spine* 1993;18:35-40.

101. Svensson HO, et al: Low-back pain in relation to other diseases and cardiovascular risk factors. *Spine* 1983;8:277-285.

102. Kelsey JL, et al: Acute prolapsed lumbar intervertebral disc: An epidemiologic study with special reference to driving automobiles and cigarette smoking. *Spine* 1984;9:608-613.

103. Leboeuf-Yde C, Kyvik KO, Bruun NH: Low back pain and lifestyle: Part I. Smoking: Information from a population-based sample of 29,424 twins. *Spine* 1998;23:2207-2214.

104. Hoogendoorn WE, et al: Systematic review of psychosocial factors at work and private life as risk factors for back pain. *Spine* 2000;25:2114-2125.

105. Kerr MS, et al: Biomechanical and psychosocial risk factors for low back pain at work. *Am J Public Health* 2001;91:1069-1075.

106. Davis KG, Heaney CA: The relationship between psychosocial work characteristics and low back pain: Underlying methodological issues. *Clin Biomech* 2000;15:389-406.

107. Svensson HO, Anderson GBJ: Low back pain in 40- to 47-year old men: Work history and work environment factors. *Spine* 1983;8:272-276.

108. Bigos SJ, et al: Back injuries in industry: A retrospective study: III. Employee-related factors. *Spine* 1986;11:252-256.

109. Spengler DM, et al: Back injuries in industry: A retrospective study. Overview and cost analysis. *Spine* 1986;11:241-245.

110. Johnston JM, et al: Stressful psychosocial work environment increases risk for back pain among retail material handlers. *Am J Ind Med* 2003;43:179-187.

111. Elfering A, et al: Time control, catecholamines and back pain among young nurses. *Scand J Work Environ Health* 2002;28:386-393.

112. Dionne CE, et al: Formal education and back pain: A review. *J Epidemiol Community Health* 2001;55:455-468.

113. Carroll LJ, Cassidy JD, Cote P: Depression as a risk factor for onset of an episode of troublesome neck and low back pain. *Pain* 2004;107:134-139.

114. Truchon M: Determinants of chronic disability related to low-back pain: Towards an integrative biopsychosocial model. *Disabil Rehabil* 2001;23:758-767.

115. Waddell G: A new clinical model for the treatment of low-back pain. *Spine* 1987;12:632-644.

116. Pincus T, et al: A systematic review of psychological factors as predictors of chronicity/disability in prospective cohorts of low back pain. *Spine* 2002;27:E109-120.

117. Wang SM, et al: Low back pain during pregnancy: Prevalence, risk factors, and outcomes. *Obstet Gynecol* 2004;104:65-70.

118. To WW, Wong MW: Factors associated with back pain symptoms in pregnancy and the persistence of pain 2 years after pregnancy. *Acta Obstet Gynecol Scand* 2003;82:1086-1091.

119. Harreby M, et al: Risk factors for low back pain in a cohort of 1389 Danish school children: An epidemiologic study. *Eur Spine J* 1999;8:444-450.

120. Balague F, et al: Non-specific low-back pain among schoolchildren: A field survey with analysis of some associated factors. *J Spinal Disord* 1994;7:374-379.

121. Jones GT, et al: Predictors of low back pain in British schoolchildren: A population-based prospective cohort study. *Pediatrics* 2003;111:822-828.

122. Limon S, Valinsky LJ, Ben-Shalom Y: Children at risk: Risk factors for low back pain in the elementary school environment. *Spine* 2004;29:697-702.

123. Negrini S, Carabalona R, Sibilla P: Backpack as a daily load for schoolchildren. *Lancet* 1999;354:1974.

124. Negrini S, Carabalona R: Backpacks on! Schoolchildren's perceptions of load, associations with back pain and factors determining the load. *Spine* 2002;27:187-195.

125. Heliovaara M, Impivaara O, et al: Lumbar disc syndrome in Finland. *J Epidemiol Community Health* 1987;41:251-258.

126. Tubach F, Beaute J, Leclerc A: Natural history and prognostic indicators of sciatica. *J Clin Epidemiol* 2004;57:174-179.

127. Balague F, Troussier B, Salminen JJ: Non-specific low back pain in children and adolescents: Risk factors. *Eur Spine J* 1999;8:429-438.

128. Indahl A: Low back pain: Diagnosis, treatment, and prognosis. *Scand J Rheumatol* 2004;33:199-209.

129. Rainville J, et al: Low back and cervical spine disorders. *Orthop Clin North Am* 1996;27:729-746.

130. Waxman R, Tennant A, Helliwell P: A prospective follow-up study of low back pain in the community. *Spine* 2000;25:2085-2090.

131. McGorry RW, et al: The relation between pain intensity, disability, and the episodic nature of chronic and recurrent low back pain. *Spine* 2000;25:834-841.

132. Roland M, Morris R: A study of the natural history of low-back pain: Part II. Development of guidelines for trials of treatment in primary care. *Spine* 1983;8:145-150.

133. Roland M, Morris R: A study of the natural history of back pain: Part I. Development of a reliable and sensitive

measure of disability in low-back pain. *Spine* 1983;8:
141-144.

134. Beutler WJ, et al: The natural history of spondylolysis and
spondylolisthesis: 45-year follow-up evaluation. *Spine*
2003;28:1027-1035.

135. Lauerman WC, Cain JE: Isthmic spondylolisthesis in the
adult. *J Am Acad Orthop Surg* 1996;4:201-208.

136. Jarvik JJ, et al: The Longitudinal Assessment of Imaging
and Disability of the Back (LAIDBack) Study: Baseline
data. *Spine* 2001;26:1158-1166.

137. Powell MC, et al: Prevalence of lumbar disc degeneration
observed by magnetic resonance in symptomless women.
Lancet 1986;8520:1366-1367.

138. Jensen MC, et al: Magnetic resonance imaging of the lumbar spine in people without back pain. *N Engl J Med*
1994;331:69-73.

139. Boden SD, Davis DO, Dina TS, Patronas NJ, Wiesel SW:
Abnormal magnetic-resonance scans of the lumbar spine
in asymptomatic subjects: A prospective investigation. *J
Bone Joint Surg Am* 1990;72:403-408.

140. Videman T, Nurminen M, Troup JD: Lumbar spinal
pathology in cadaveric material in relation to history of
back pain, occupation, and physical loading. *Spine*
1990;15:728-740.

141. Videman T, et al: Associations between back pain history
and lumbar MRI findings. *Spine* 2003;28:582-588.

142. Freemont AJ, et al: Nerve ingrowth into diseased intervertebral disc in chronic back pain. *Lancet* 1997;9072:178-
181.

143. Moneta GB, et al: Reported pain during lumbar discography as a function of anular ruptures and disc degenera-

tion: A re-analysis of 833 discograms. *Spine* 1994;19:1968-
1974.

144. Saifuddin A, et al: The value of lumbar spine magnetic
resonance imaging in the demonstration of anular tears.
Spine 1998;23:453-457.

145. Vergauwen S, et al: Distribution and incidence of degenerative spine changes in patients with a lumbo-sacral transitional vertebra. *Eur Spine J* 1997;6:168-172.

146. Wigh R, Anthony HJ: Transitional lumbosacral discs:
Probability of herniation. *Spine* 1981;6:168-171.

147. O'Driscoll C, Irwin A, Saifuddin A: Variations in morphology of the lumbosacral junction on sagittal MRI:
Correlation with plain radiography. *Skeletal Radiol*
1996;25:225-230.

148. Hahn P, Strobel J, Hahn F: Verification of lumbosacral
segments on MR images: Identification of transitional
vertebrae. *Radiology* 1992;182:580-581.

149. Peh W, Siu T, Chan J: Determining the lumbar vertebral
segments on magnetic resonance imaging. *Spine*
1999;24:1852-1855.

150. MacGibbon B, Farfan H: A radiologic survey of various
configurations of the lumbar spine. *Spine* 1979;4:168-171.

151. Castellvi A, Goldstein L, Chan D: Lumbosacral transitional vertebrae and their relationship with lumbar
extradural defects. *Spine* 1989;9:493-495.

152. Elster A: Bertolotti's syndrome revisited: Transitional vertebrae of the lumbar spine. *Spine* 1989;14:1373-1377.

153. Luoma K, et al: Lumbosacral transitional vertebra. *Spine*
2004;29:200-205.

154. Waddell G, McCulloch JA, Kummel E, Venner RM:
Nonorganic physical signs in low-back pain. *Spine*
1980;5:117-125.

CHAPTER 3

NONSURGICAL MANAGEMENT OF LOW BACK PAIN

JAMES RAINVILLE, MD
CAROL HARTIGAN, MD
REILLY KEFFER, DO

Low back pain (LBP) of musculoskeletal etiology is reported by 75% of all adults at some point in their lives and has a point prevalence in the adult population of approximately 20%.[1,2] Most persons with LBP manage their symptoms independently; only one third of adults with LBP actually seek medical care for their symptoms.[3-5] For about 4% of the population, LBP is a chronic problem, and these individuals frequently seek medical care, often from multiple providers.[5,6] In total, LBP consumes an extraordinary amount of medical care resources per year, most of which is nonsurgical.

Nonsurgical care of LBP can be viewed as managing the natural history of the disorder to ensure that function is recovered as quickly as possible while symptoms are adequately controlled. Therefore, the delivery of nonsurgical care for LBP requires an understanding of current theories about its causes and its natural history. When these are understood, the essential components of treatment fall into place, including patient education, modalities used for symptom control, and the management of resultant disability.

ETIOLOGY OF LOW BACK PAIN

Many spine specialists currently consider a degenerative etiology for most LBP, in which progressive degeneration of the intervertebral disks and facet joints periodically produces pain in some individuals through the influence of degeneration, secondary inflammation, and nociception.[7]

For decades, the injury model has been used to explain spinal degeneration and most episodes of LBP because it was believed that structures in the spine deteriorated secondary to the deleterious effects of environmental and occupational exposures. However, epidemiologic studies report only limited evidence to support the injury theory. Less than 2% of the variance in reported back pain can be attributed to physical exposures to activities such as whole body vibrations or frequent lifting.[8,9]

Clearly, environmental and physical exposures are not the causes of most LBP. Various ergonomic and educational interventions inspired by the injury model, which attempt to reduce the risk of injury through altered body mechanics and decreased exposure to activities that stress the back, have met with limited success.[10]

Over the last decade, our understanding of the causes of spinal degeneration has improved; evidence now suggests that degeneration results from genetically predetermined and age-related loss of cellular function within the joints of the spine. In the late 1980s and early 1990s, several authors reported that disk degeneration and herniations often clustered in families.[11,12] These reports were followed by studies of cohorts of twins, which reported that 74% of the variance observed in disk degeneration on lumbar MRI scans was predicted by heritability, with environment and exposures accounting for only a tiny amount of the variance.[13,14] In addition to genetic susceptibility to spinal degeneration, evidence suggests that the development of LBP in the presence of degeneration also may be strongly influenced by genetic factors that affect pain sensitivity.[15,16] These discoveries have significant implications in terms of patient education. Because genetically predetermined factors appear to be the major cause of spinal degeneration, patients do not need to avoid physical activities as a mechanism to prevent further degeneration and pain. Educating patients about these findings can reduce their fear about activities causing further injury or harm and help them understand that return to normal activities, including exercise, is safe and without major influence on the risk for future back pain.[17]

NATURAL HISTORY OF LOW BACK PAIN

Although LBP is one of the most common and unpleasant human afflictions, the prognosis for recovery is quite favorable. Within 1 month of onset, most patients experience substantial reduction in pain intensity and disability, and often return to work, regardless of treatment.[18,19] Patients should be educated about this favorable prognosis. Because therapeutic modalities have demonstrated little consistent ability to favorably impact the natural history of LBP, most interventions for acute LBP should be viewed as efforts to minimize the symptoms and disability while spontaneous improvement occurs.

Although the short-term prognosis is excellent, many patients have persistent minor symptoms and report mild residual disability 1 year after an acute episode,[18,20] and up to 60% will report recurrent episodes of acute LBP over the next year.[21,22] Most recurrences are minor in intensity, with only half requiring additional medical attention and less than one third resulting in work-related disability.[23] Current data suggest that recurrence rates are not influenced by the type of health care provider for the initial episode, nor are they increased in patients who remain physically active.[24,25] Educating patients about these findings can be helpful in preventing discouragement when LBP recurs, for promoting self-care for future episodes, and for encouraging continued physical function.

The prognosis is less favorable for patients who present with chronic LBP; about two thirds will still have pain at 3-year follow-up.[26] Fortunately, most maintain employment and modest levels of function despite their symptoms.[27] For this group, therapeutic efforts usually focus on minimizing the impact of LBP on daily function.

In summary, LBP is a dynamic process, with high rates for incidence, recurrence, and recovery. Nonsurgical care of back pain is best viewed as an effort to help patients manage their predicament when they are at their worst as opposed to curing them of this affliction.

SYMPTOM MANAGEMENT

Symptom management, which is the major focus of most LBP-related medical encounters, takes many forms, including patient education, medications, modalities, exercise, and alternative therapies. In this section, we will review specific categories of medical interventions in terms of their effectiveness for the treatment of LBP.

Medications

Oral Anti-Inflammatory Medications

Nonsteroidal anti-inflammatory drugs (NSAIDs) are a standard first-line drug treatment for back pain and are prescribed by primary care physicians for two thirds of patients with LBP.[28] NSAIDs are prescribed for their analgesic actions and to treat presumed inflammation. Two recent systematic reviews of more than 50 randomized controlled trials of nonselective NSAIDs concluded that NSAIDs are more effective than placebo in treating acute LBP, although no one specific NSAID was deemed superior over others.[29,30]

The efficacy of NSAIDs for chronic LBP is less clear. In the review by van Tulder and associates[29] in 2000, both the scarcity of studies examining this issue and the design of the studies did not permit any evidence-based recommendations on the effectiveness of NSAIDs in patients with chronic LBP. However, a recent study suggests that rofecoxib may have a slight advantage over placebo at the 4-week period, but long-term follow-up was not reported.[31] It should be noted that as of this writing, rofecoxib has been withdrawn from the world market as a result of increased risk of adverse cardiovascular events.

Use of NSAIDs to treat sciatica has received limited study. It is known that high levels of inflammatory mediators are present in acute disk herniations, but the levels of these mediators has not correlated with the intensity of sciatica or the severity of findings on clinical examination.[32] Several authors have reported some advantage of NSAIDs for sciatic pain, but more research clearly is needed in this area.[33,34]

Some patients respond differently to various NSAIDs; therefore, some clinicians will try several alternative NSAIDs for patients who do not initially respond to treatment. Gastrointestinal, renal, and cardiac side effects are not uncommon, and important consideration must be given to these risks when prescribing this class of medications, particularly in the elderly.

Oral Steroids

Some clinicians use a brief course of oral steroids to treat acute, severe LBP or sciatica. Authors of the only study of oral steroids we found reported that dexamethasone was not superior to placebo for treating lumbosacral radicular pain, although more rapid improvement in straight leg raising was noted in the steroid group.[35]

Muscle Relaxants

Muscle relaxants have no direct peripheral action on muscles. Although the mechanism of action of these medications is not completely understood, their effect is known to be secondary to action within the central nervous system. Muscle relaxants are widely used in the treatment of supposed muscle spasms associated with acute LBP, with between one and two thirds of patients receiving these medications from primary care providers.[28,38] A recent systematic review of 30 randomized and/or double-blinded controlled trials on the use of muscle relaxants reported that muscle relaxants are more effective than placebo in providing short-term pain relief (limited to within the first week) for patients with acute LBP.[36,37] Evidence to advocate their use for patients with chronic LBP is insufficient, and evidence of their utility in sciatica is nonexistent.[37] Because the use of muscle relaxants is not associated with more rapid functional recovery, their clinical effectiveness is marginal at best.[38]

Muscle relaxants are no more effective than NSAIDs alone, and no additional benefit is gained when using a muscle relaxant in combination with an NSAID. Moreover, muscle relaxants have the potential for producing sedation, tolerance, withdrawal symptoms, and addiction. Therefore, these medications must be used cautiously during only the first weeks of acute LBP, if used at all.

Analgesics

Analgesics, or medications that are able to reduce pain, would be a logical choice for treatment of LBP symptoms. Unfortunately, they have received only limited study. Acetaminophen is the most widely available over-the-counter analgesic, but it is recommended by primary care providers to only 4% of patients with acute LBP.[28] We were unable to identify any studies of its efficacy for this disorder. Narcotic analgesics are prescribed to approximately 12% of patients with acute LBP.[28] This low percentage suggests that most patients with acute LBP are successfully managed without these medications, although some patients with severe symptoms may benefit from a brief course of narcotic analgesics.

For chronic LBP, the use of narcotic analgesics is both common and controversial. Several studies suggest that they are efficacious for a selected group of patients. Tramadol, a compound with weak opioid activity and adjuvant analgesic properties, was reported to modestly reduce pain compared with placebo in one randomized, controlled trial and also was reported to be effective when combined with acetaminophen in another.[39,40] Jamison and associates[41] reported that opioid therapy had a positive effect on pain intensity and mood, but little effect on activity or sleep. It should be noted that most patients with chronic LBP neither request nor desire narcotic analgesics. Authors of a study comparing patients who used NSAIDs with those prescribed opioids for chronic LBP reported that opioid use was not predicted by pain intensity or clinical findings, but instead by age, depression, personality disorder, and history of substance abuse.[42]

Injections

Trigger Point Injections

Myofascial trigger points are frequently diagnosed in a variety of musculoskeletal disorders, including acute and chronic LBP. The diagnosis of trigger points remains controversial, and reproducibility of trigger point diagnosis between different examiners has been reported to be unreliable.[43] Authors of recent reviews of needling therapies in the management of trigger points reported that the nature of the injected substance (ie, lidocaine, normal saline, steroid, etc) did not affect the outcome,[44,45] and they reported that wet needling was not superior to dry needling of the trigger point. It is still unclear to what extent the efficacy of trigger point injections exceeds that of the placebo response.

Facet Joint Injection

The facet joints have long been considered a significant source of pain in patients with chronic LBP; however, the prevalence, diagnosis, and efficacy of treatment with injections are controversial. There is a wide disparity in estimates of the prevalence of so-called facet joint syndrome, with a general consensus that occurrence is increased in the elderly population. The different theories that propose mechanisms for pain generation by the facet joints remain unproved. Lumbar facet joint osteoarthritis is observed radiographically in many asymptomatic individuals; however, despite suggestions that severely degenerated joints are more likely to be symptomatic, radiographic findings alone are inadequate for a specific diagnosis.[46,47] Nothing in the history or physical examination is pathognomonic for diagnosis of facet joint syndrome.[48,49] At this time, the only reliable way to make the diagnosis requires documenting defined periods of pain relief following fluoroscopically guided local anesthetic blocks of the joint itself or its corresponding nerve supply.[49]

Lumbar facet joint mediated pain is treated by either intra-articular injection with corticosteroid or percutaneous ablation of the nerve supply to the joints. However, the efficacy of these interventions is much debated. In a recent review, Slipman and associates[50] reported that available evidence for the treatment of facet joint

syndrome with intra-articular injections is level III (moderate) to level IV (limited), and the treatment response in a controlled trial was marginal.[51] Evidence for the use of radiofrequency denervation of facet joints is moderate.[50] The design and outcomes of trials studying the efficacy of these treatments of facet joint syndrome vary considerably, and additional well-designed, high-quality, prospective, randomized controlled trials are needed.

Epidural Steroid Injections

In recent years, epidural steroid injections have gained popularity in the treatment of patients with disk herniations and radiculopathies. Various studies have documented the inflammatory reaction following disk herniations.[32,52] Locally applied corticosteroids seem to be a logical choice for treatment of this type of inflammation because of their effect on membrane stabilization and antinociceptive C-fibers and their interference with neuropeptide and inflammatory mediator activities.[53]

Although epidural steroid injections have long been used in the treatment of LBP and radicular symptoms attributed to disk herniation, controversy as to their efficacy continues, with the literature characterized by conflicting results. Koes and associates,[54] in a systematic review of 15 randomized clinical trials evaluating the use of epidural steroid injections in patients with LBP and sciatica, noted that about half of the studies reported positive outcomes, whereas the other half reported negative outcomes. The authors concluded that the efficacy of these injections remains to be established and that, if anything, the benefits are of short duration.[54] Weinstein and Herring[55] reported a wide variation in the techniques and procedures of epidural steroid application. Because fluoroscopically guided injections were not used in any studies prior to 2000,[55] results of needle misplacements with blind injection techniques may be compared with those of verified needle placement using fluoroscopic guidance with contrast enhancement.[56,57] Although the authors[55] lamented that the number of quality trials was limited and that significant methodologic flaws were noted in the studies reviewed, they concluded that fair evidence supports lumbar epidural steroid injections for the treatment of sciatica associated with disk herniation. Epidural steroid injections appear to produce a short-term (several weeks) reduction of leg pain; however, these injections do not alter long-term outcomes, including the need for spine surgery,[58] nor do they appreciably change functional outcomes. Clinicians who decide to use epidural steroid injections must consider the limited effectiveness of this procedure in the context of the severity of symptoms, the favorable natural history of this problem, and the cost of this intervention.

Bed Rest and Activity Advice

Occasionally, acute LBP or sciatica can be so severe that a patient reports the inability to tolerate being out of bed. In these circumstances, brief bed rest can be sanctioned, but evidence suggests that even these patients should be advised to get out of bed as soon as possible and as much as possible. In general, bed rest has been found to have no positive therapeutic effects in the treatment of LBP or sciatica, and advised bed rest has been found to increase disability and work loss.[59,60] When advised bed rest was compared with advice to resume normal activities as tolerated, bed rest offered no clinical advantage, and patients advised to resume usual activities reported less lost work time and disability.[61,62] Delivering the message that it is safe to remain active with acute LBP positively affects outcome.

Advice to increase activities is also useful for patients with subacute LBP. Advice to avoid guarding, to perform normal activities, to avoid being "careful," to walk normally, to remain active through episodes of stabbing pain, to lift everyday objects using the back, and to use caution only when lifting heavy objects resulted in significantly less work absence at 7-month and 5-year follow-up compared with standard medical care in one study.[63,64]

Physical Therapy Modalities

Cold and Heat

Many patients with LBP seek and use simple modalities to reduce their discomfort. Surprisingly, the effectiveness of ice, which is one of the most common available modalities, in reducing pain, inflammation, and disability in acute LBP never has been reported specifically. Ice, applied several times a day for several days, has been reported to reduce inflammation and disability in acute ankle sprains,[65] and ice has been reported to increase the pain threshold without the negative sedating effect of heat.[66,67] Because some patients temporarily feel better after using ice, instruction in self-application may be

useful. The simplicity of self-application of ice makes it difficult to justify its application in the costly therapeutic setting.

The local application of heat is another commonly used, self-administered modality for LBP. Its effectiveness, however, is not clearly established, and evidence to support or refute its use is insufficient.[68,69] Several studies of patients with acute and subacute LBP report worse outcomes at 3 months in patients receiving regular heat treatment.[70-72] Two small studies of patients with acute LBP reported marginally improved pain scores at the 5-day follow-up in patients who applied a heat wrap for 8 hours a day for 3 days compared with patients receiving an oral placebo; however, outcomes beyond 5 days were not reported.[73,74] Heat should be applied judiciously because it may aggravate the inflammatory response in the first few days after injury, and it produces sedation. In the initial stages of active mobilization, some authors believe that application of heat before one or two treatments may facilitate stretch and reduce pain; however, this remains unproved. Because heat may be self-applied, it is difficult to justify its regular application in outpatient therapy.

Electrical Stimulation

Transcutaneous electrical nerve stimulation (TENS) presumably is used to reduce pain by electrically stimulating peripheral nerves with skin electrodes. In 1994, Herman and associates[75] reported no differences between work-injured patients with subacute LBP undergoing exercise treatment with true TENS and those receiving placebo TENS for pain, disability, and functional outcomes. A recent meta-analysis of the efficacy of TENS for chronic LBP evaluated five randomized controlled trials and demonstrated no evidence to support the use of TENS for LBP.[76] The authors noted inconsistency in type, site, duration, frequency, and intensity of TENS application between the studies.

Traction

Traction often is applied in outpatient therapy, based on the theory that distraction of the vertebrae might reduce LBP or leg pain attributed to compression. Manual traction, autotraction (patient exerts force), gravitational traction (suspension device), or motorized traction may be applied. Outpatient traction often is complemented by other empirically applied physical therapy treatments.

Two reviews of the literature on the application of outpatient traction reported that poor methodology precluded drawing any conclusion regarding its efficacy.[77,78]

Manipulation and Mobilization

Manipulation and mobilization have been and remain popular treatments for LBP. Though relatively safe, the effectiveness of such treatments is marginal at best. Several studies have reported no differences in outcomes for patients with acute and subacute LBP treated with chiropractic manipulation or manual therapy and patients treated with physical therapy.[79-81] One study reported that manual therapy resulted in outcomes only marginally better than the outcomes for patients who received the minimal intervention of an educational booklet.[79] Two studies reported no statistically significant difference for patients with subacute and chronic LBP treated with osteopathic manipulation or chiropractic manual care and patients assigned to standard medical care.[82,83] Another study reported no differences in outcome between trunk strengthening exercises combined with spinal manipulative therapy and trunk strengthening exercises combined with NSAIDs.[84] Traditional Finnish bone-setting led to modestly greater improvements in Oswestry Disability Scores compared to exercise therapy and physical therapy.[85] A 2004 review of the efficacy of spinal manipulation and mobilization for LBP reported few other studies of good methodologic quality for evaluation.[86]

Numerous physical examination maneuvers, in combination with pain purported to detect sacroiliac joint dysfunction, have been reported to have poor inter- and intrarater reliability,[87] and they are positive in 20% of the asymptomatic population.[88] Studies examining manual therapy interventions for presumed sacroiliac joint dysfunction have been based on these unreliable history and physical examination maneuvers.[89] Furthermore, roentgen stereophotogrammetric analysis following presumed sacroiliac joint manipulation demonstrates that the position of the sacrum in relation to the ilium is unaltered by treatment.[90]

Exercise

Various exercises, ranging from simple to complex and nonspecific to specific, commonly are used in the treatment of LBP. For decades, floor exercise programs have advocated trunk flexion and/or extension movements and lower extremity stretches (pelvic tilt, knee to chest, bridging, rotating the legs, hamstring stretch, superman). However, these exercises largely are applied inconsistently and heterogeneously. In the 1980s, programs were developed to classify patients according to physical examination results and then recommend exercises based on their classification.[91,92] Unfortunately, the reliability of classification was poor.[93] In the late 1980s more rigorous floor exercise programs, which focused on trunk strength and control, were introduced and included the exercise ball, but no controlled trials have evaluated this method, known as dynamic lumbar stabilization.[94] Since then, dynamic lumbar stabilization programs have evolved. Core strengthening programs, based on more challenging multiplane trunk focused exercises, are currently popular.[95] Many contemporary programs, including Pilates and various yoga programs, use core strengthening principles and exercises. No literature specifically evaluates these programs or documents superiority over simple single-plane trunk strengthening performed on resisted health club equipment.[95] However, the use of exercise as a treatment for back pain has been studied in patients with acute, subacute, and chronic back pain with mixed results.

Acute Low Back Pain

Unfortunately, few studies on the effectiveness of exercises for acute LBP qualify as high quality.[96,97] Several studies regarded as high quality compare flexion and extension exercises for acute LBP with other nonsurgical treatments, including sham ultrasound, standard care, bed rest, no intervention, and advice to remain active as tolerated. None of these studies reported evidence that exercise was harmful, increased back pain, or resulted in superior outcomes.[59,62,98,99]

Subacute and Recurrent Low Back Pain

Exercise may have greater value for the treatment of persistent and recurrent LBP. Significant improvement in return to work and significantly less work absence over 2 years was reported in a group of patients with subacute back injury who underwent a graded, nonpain-contingent exercise program when compared to controls.[72] This outcome may have resulted from a reduction in the frequency or severity of recurrent episodes of pain or from greater tendency to self-treat with exercise in patients who received past instruction.[101,102]

Chronic Low Back Pain

In a systematic review of the evidence, van Tulder and associates[102] reported that exercise may help patients with chronic LBP return to normal activities and work. Additionally, exercise is safe for individuals with LBP and does not increase the risk of future back injuries or work absence.[17] Substantial evidence supports the use of exercise as a means of improving back flexibility and strength and of reducing pain, and exercise can reduce the behavioral, cognitive, and disability aspects associated with LBP.[17]

Acupuncture and Massage

Acupuncture is based on the assumption that disruptions of optimal patterns of energy flow may result in pain and purportedly are corrected by needle stimulation of specific points close to the skin. A National Institutes of Health consensus conference on acupuncture reported that acupuncture studies were, for the most part, poorly designed, of inadequate sample size, and lacking control groups.[103] For the same reasons, more specific reviews of acupuncture as treatment for LBP also report inability to conclude effectiveness or ineffectiveness of this intervention.[104,105] One recent study randomized chronic LBP patients to receive traditional Chinese medical acupuncture (10 visits), therapeutic massage (10 visits), or self-care educational materials.[106] At 10 weeks, the massage group had superior symptom relief and function compared with the self-care and acupuncture groups. At 1 year, however, no difference between the massage and self-care groups was reported for symptoms and function, but the outcomes of the massage group remained superior to the acupuncture outcomes.[106]

CONCLUSIONS

Nonsurgical management of LBP consists mainly of managing the natural history of this disorder and controlling pain while helping patients to remain as functional as possible. Nonsurgical management should always include patient education about the cause of spinal degeneration, the periodic association of degeneration and symptoms, and the favorable natural history of these disorders. Patients should be advised to stay active during and after an episode of LBP, because doing so may hasten recovery and does not increase the risk for further degeneration and pain. This simple advice consumes only minutes of office time and may have significant impact on outcomes.

Many modalities are available to aid physicians in treating LBP, with short-term use of medications offering limited benefit for some patients. Injections of corticosteroids may offer some short-term benefits for selected patients with sciatica and others with hard to define facet syndromes. Ice may be the most easily applied and inexpensive physical therapy modality available for the treatment of acute LBP, although its efficacy is not proved. Various labor intensive and expensive physical modalities and manipulative techniques have received some study, but none has withstood rigorous research. Exercise appears to have value for improving function in patients with recurrent or chronic LBP, but its usefulness in acute pain is not clearly established.

In general, with the current lack of well-proved treatments for LBP, clinicians should keep their treatment simple and project a positive attitude to reinforce the safety and importance of patients remaining functional.

REFERENCES

1. Heliovaara M, Sievers K, Impivaara O, et al: Descriptive epidemiology and public health aspects of low back pain. *Ann Med* 1989;21:327-333.

2. Smedley J, Inskip H, Cooper C, Coggon D: Natural history of low back pain: A longitudinal study in nurses. *Spine* 1998;23:2422-2426.

3. Cares TS, Evans AT, Hadler NM, et al: Acute severe low back pain: A population-based study of prevalence and care-seeking. *Spine* 1996;21:339-344.

4. Cote P, Casssidy JD, Carroll L: The treatment of neck and low back pain: Who seeks care? Who goes where? *Med Care* 2001;39:956-967.

5. Ijzenberg W, Burdorf A: Patterns of care for low back pain in a working population. *Spine* 2004;29:1362-1368.

6. Cares TS, Evans A, Hadler N, Kalsbeek W, McLaughlin C, Fryer J: Care-seeking among individuals with chronic low back pain. *Spine* 1995;20:312-317.

7. Weinstein JN: A 45-year-old man with low back pain and a numb left foot. *JAMA* 1998;280:730-736.

8. Damkot DK, Pope MH, Lord J, Frymoyer JW: The relationship between work history, work environment, and low-back pain in men. *Spine* 1984;9:395-399.

9. Levangie PK: Association of low back pain with self-reported risk factors among patients seeking physical therapy services. *Phys Ther* 1999;79:757-766.

10. Leclaire R, Esdaile JM, Suissa S, Rossignol M, Proulx R, Dupuis M: Back school in a first episode of compensated acute low back pain: A clinical trial to assess efficacy and prevent relapse. *Arch Phys Med Rehabil* 1996;77:673-679.

11. Matsui H, Terahata N, Tsuji H, Hirano N, Naruse Y: Familial predisposition and clustering for juvenile lumbar disc herniation. *Spine* 1992;17:1323-1328.

12. Postacchini F, Lami R, Pugliese O: Familial predisposition to discogenic low-back pain: An epidemiologic and immunogenetic study. *Spine* 1988;12:1403-1406.

13. Battie MC, Videman T, Gibbons LE, Fisher LD, Manninen H, Gill K: Determinants of lumbar degeneration: A study relating lifetime exposures and magnetic resonance imaging findings in identical twins. *Spine* 1995;20:2601-2612.

14. Sambrook PN, MacGregor AJ, Spector TD: Genetic influences on cervical and lumbar disc degeneration: A magnetic resonance imaging study of twins. *Arthritis Rheum* 1999;42:366-372.

15. Bengtsson B, Thorson J: Backpain: A study of twins. *Acta Genet Med Gemellol (Roma)* 1991;40:83-90.

16. MacGregor AJ, Andrew T, Sambrook PN, Spector TD: Structural, psychological, and genetic influences on low back and neck pain: A study of adult female twins. *Arthritis Rheum* 2004;51:160-167.

17. Rainville J, Hartigan C, Martinez E, Limke J, Jouve C, Finno M: Exercise as a treatment for chronic low back pain. *Spine J* 2004;4:106-115.

18. Von Korff M, Saunders K: The course of back pain in primary care. *Spine* 1996;21:2833-2837.

19. Pengel LH, Herbert RD, Maher CG, Refshauge KM: Acute low back pain: Systematic review of its prognosis. *BMJ* 2003;337:323-325.

20. Croft PR, Macfarlane GJ, Papageorgiou AC, Thomas D, Silman AJ: Outcome of low back pain in general practice: A prospective study. *BMJ* 1998;316:1356-1359.

21. Hestbaek L, Leboeuf-Yde C, Manniche C: Low back pain: What is the long-term course? A review of studies of general patient populations. *Eur Spine J* 2003;12:149-165.

22. Elder LA, Burdorf A: Prevalence, incidence, and recurrence of low back pain in scaffolders during a 3-year follow-up study. *Spine* 2004;29:E101-E106.

23. Wasiak R, Pransky G, Verma S, Webster B: Recurrence of low back pain: Definition-sensitivity analysis using administrative data. *Spine* 2003;28:2283-2291.

24. Carey TS, Garrett JM, Jackson A, Hadler N: Recurrence and care seeking after acute back pain: Results of a long-term follow-up study. North Carolina Back Pain Project. *Med Care* 1999;37:157-164.

25. Hagen KB, Hilde G, Jamtvedt G, Winnem MF: The Cochrane review of advice to stay active as a single treatment for low back pain and sciatica. *Spine* 2002;27:1736-1741.

26. Smith BH, Elliot AM, Hannaford PC, Chambers WA, Smith WC: Factors related to the onset and persistence of chronic back pain in the community: Results from a general population study. *Spine* 2004;29:1032-1040.

27. Carey TS, Garrett JM, Jackman AM: Beyond the good prognosis: Examination of an inception cohort of patients with chronic low back pain. *Spine* 2000;25:115-120.

28. Cherkin DC, Wheeler KJ, Barlow W, Deyo RA: Medication use for low back pain in primary care. *Spine* 1998;23:607-614.

29. van Tulder MW, Scholten RJ, Koes BW, Deyo RA: Nonsteroidal anti-inflammatory drugs for low back pain: A systematic review within the framework of the Cochrane Collaboration Back Review Group. *Spine* 2000;25:2501-2513.

30. Schnitzer TJ, Ferraro A, Hunsche E, Kong SX: A comprehensive review of clinical trials on the efficacy and safety of drugs for the treatment of low back pain. *J Pain Symptom Manage* 2004;28:72-95.

31. Katz N, Ju WD, Krupa DA, et al: Efficacy and safety of rofecoxib in patients with chronic low back pain: Results from two 4-week, randomized, placebo-controlled, parallel-group, double-blind trials. *Spine* 2003;28:851-858.

32. Piperno M, Hellio le Graverand MP, Reboul P, et al: Phospholipase A2 activity in herniated lumbar discs: Clinical correlations and inhibition by piroxicam. *Spine* 1997;22:2061-2065.

33. Hatori M, Kokubun S: Clinical use of etodolac for the treatment of lumbar disc herniation. *Curr Med Res Opin* 1999;15:193-201.

34. Dreiser RL, Le Parc JM, Velicitat P, Lleu PL: Oral meloxicam is effective in acute sciatica: Two randomised, double-blind trials versus placebo or diclofenac. *Inflamm Res* 2001;50(suppl 1):S17-S23.

35. Haimovic IC, Beresford HR: Dexamethasone is not superior to placebo for treating lumbosacral radicular pain. *Neurology* 1986;36:1593-1594.

36. Browning R, Jackson JL, O'Malley PG: Cyclobenzaprine and back pain: A meta-analysis. *Arch Intern Med* 2001;161:1613-1620.

37. van Tulder MW, Touray T, Furlan AD, Solway S, Bouter LM: Muscle relaxants for nonspecific low back pain: A systematic review within the framework of the Cochrane collaboration. *Spine* 2003;28:1978-1992.

38. Bernstein E, Carey TS, Garrett JM: The use of muscle relaxant medications in acute low back pain. *Spine* 2004;29:1346-1351.

39. Schnitzer TJ, Gray WL, Paster RZ, Kamin M: Efficacy of tramadol in treatment of chronic low back pain. *J Rheumatol* 2000;27:772-778.

40. Ruoff GE, Rosenthal N, Jordon D, Karim R, Ramin M: Tramadol/acetaminophen combination tablets for the

treatment of chronic lower back pain: A multicenter, randomized, double-blind, placebo-controlled outpatient study. *Clin Ther* 2003;25:1123-1141.

41. Jamison RN, Raymond SA, Slawsby EZ, Nedeljkovic SS, Katz NP: Opioid therapy for chronic noncancer back pain: A randomized prospective study. *Spine* 1998;23:2591-2600.

42. Breckenridge J, Clark JD: Patient characteristics associated with opioid verses nonsteroidal anti-inflammatory drug management of chronic low back pain. *J Pain* 2003;4:344-350.

43. Gerwin RD, Shannon S, Hong C, Hubbard D, Gevirtz R: Interrater reliability in myofascial trigger point examination. *Pain* 1997;69:65-73.

44. Cummings TM, White AR: Needling therapies in the management of myofascial trigger point pain: A systematic review. *Arch Phys Med Rehabil* 2001;82:986-992.

45. Garvey TA, Marks MR, Wiesel SW: A prospective, randomized, double-blind evaluation of trigger-point injection therapy for low back pain. *Pain* 1989;14:962-964.

46. Schwarzer AC, Aprill CN, Derby R, Fortin J, Kine G, Bogduk N: The relative contributions of the disc and zygapophyseal joint in chronic low back pain. *Spine* 1994;19:801-806.

47. Weishaupt D, Zanetti M, Hodler J, Boos N: MR imaging of the lumbar spine: Prevalence of intervertebral disc extrusion and sequestration, nerve root compression, end plate abnormalities, and osteoarthritis of the facet joints in asymptomatic volunteers. *Radiology* 1998;209:661-666.

48. Jackson RP, Jacobs RR, Montesano PX: Facet joint injection in low-back pain: A prospective statistical study. *Spine* 1988;13:966-971.

49. Dreyfuss PH, Dreyer SJ: Lumbar zygapophysial (facet) joint injections. *Spine J* 2003;3:50S-59S.

50. Slipman WS, Bhat AL, Gilchrist RV, Isaac Z, Chou L, Lenrow DA: A critical review of the evidence for the use of zygapophysial injections and radiofrequency denervation in the treatment of low back pain. *Spine J* 2003;3:310-316.

51. Carette S, Marcoux S, Truchon R, et al: A controlled trial of corticosteroid injections into the facet joints for chronic low back pain. *N Engl J Med* 1991;325:1002-1007.

52. Takahashi H, Suguro T, Okazima Y, Motegi M, Okada Y, Kakiuchi T: Inflammatory cytokines in the herniated disc of the lumbar spine. *Spine* 1996;21:218-224.

53. Johansson A, Hao J, Sjolund B. Local corticosteroid application blocks transmission in normal nociceptive C-fibers. *Acta Anaesthesiol Scand* 1990;34:335-338.

54. Koes BW, Scholten RJ, Mens JM, Bouter LM: Epidural steroid injections for low back pain and sciatica: An updated systematic review of randomized clinical trials. *Pain Digest* 1999;9:241-247.

55. Weinstein SM, Herring, SA: Lumbar epidural steroid injections. *Spine J* 2003;3(suppl):37S-44S.

56. Mehta M, Salmon N: Extradural block: Confirmation of the injection site by X-ray monitoring. *Anaesthesia* 1985;40:1009-1012.

57. Renfrew DL, Moore TE, Kathol MH, el-Khoury GY, Lemke JH, Walker CW: Correct placement of epidural steroid injections: Fluoroscopic guidance and contrast administration. *Am J Neuroradiol* 1991;12:1003-1007.

58. Karppinen J, Malmivaara A, Kurunlahti M, et al: Periradicular infiltration for sciatica: A randomized controlled trial. *Spine* 2001;26:1059-1067.

59. Gilbert JR, Taylor DW, Hildebrand A, Evans C: Clinical trial of common treatments for low back pain in family practice. *BMJ* 1985;291:791-794.

60. Deyo RA, Diehl AK, Rosenthal M: How many days of bed rest for acute low back pain? A randomized clinical trial. *N Engl J Med* 1986;315:1064-1070.

61. Rozenberg S, Delval C, Rezvani Y, et al: Bed rest or normal activity for patients with acute low back pain: A randomized controlled trial. *Spine* 2002;14:1487-1493.

62. Malmivaara A, Hakkinen U, Aro T, et al: The treatment of acute low back pain: Bed rest, exercises, or ordinary activity? *N Engl J Med* 1995;332:351-355.

63. Indahl A, Velund L, Reikeraas O: Good prognosis for low back pain when left untampered: A randomized clinical trial. *Spine* 1995;20:473-477.

64. Indahl A, Haldorsen EH, Holm S, Reikeras O, Ursin H: Five-year follow-up study of a controlled clinical trial using light mobilization and an informative approach to low back pain. *Spine* 1998;23:2625-2630.

65. Hocutt JE Jr, Jaffe R, Rylander CR, Beebe JK: Cryotherapy in ankle sprains. *Am J Sports Med* 1982;10:316-319.

66. McMaster WC: A literary review on ice therapy in injuries. *Am J Sports Med* 1977;5:124-126.

67. McMaster WC, Liddle S, Waugh TR: Laboratory evaluation of various cold therapy modalities. *Am J Sports Med* 1978;6:291-294.

68. van Tulder MW, Koes BW, Bouter LM: Conservative treatment of acute and chronic nonspecific low back pain: A systematic review of randomized controlled trials of the most common interventions. *Spine* 1997;22:2128-2156.

69. Nordin M, Campello M: Physical therapy: Exercises and the modalities. When, what, and why? *Neurol Clin* 1999;17:75-89.

70. Mitchell RI, Carmen GM: Results of a multicenter trial using an intensive active exercise program for the treatment of acute soft tissue and back injuries. *Spine* 1990;15:514-521.

71. Lindstrom I, Ohlund C, Eek C, Wallin L, Peterson LE, Nachemson A: Mobility, strength, and fitness after a graded activity program for patients with subacute low

back pain: A randomized prospective clinical study with a behavioral therapy approach. *Spine* 1992;17:641-652.

72. Lindstrom I, Ohlund C, Eek C, et al: The effect of graded activity on patients with subacute low back pain: A randomized prospective clinical study with an operant-conditioning behavioral approach. *Phys Ther* 1992;72:279-290.

73. Nadler SF, Steiner DJ, Erasala GN, Hengehold DA, Abeln SB, Weingand KW: Continuous low-level heatwrap therapy for treating acute nonspecific low back pain. *Arch Phys Med Rehabil* 2003;84:329-334.

74. Nadler SF, Steiner DJ, Petty SR, Erasala GN, Hengehold DA, Weingand KW: Overnight use of continuous low-level heatwrap therapy for relief of low back pain. *Arch Phys Med Rehabil* 2003;84:335-342.

75. Herman E, Williams R, Stratford P, Fargas-Babjak A, Trott M: A randomized controlled trial of transcutaneous electrical nerve stimulation (CODETRON) to determine its benefits in a rehabilitation program for acute occupational low back pain. *Spine* 1994;19:561-568.

76. Brosseau L, Milne S, Robinson V, et al: Efficacy of the transcutaneous electrical nerve stimulation for the treatment of chronic low back pain: A meta-analysis. *Spine* 2002;27:596-603.

77. van der Heijden GJ, Beurskens AJ, Koes BW, Assendelft WJ, de Vet HC, Bouter LM: The efficacy of traction for back and neck pain: A systematic, blinded review of randomized clinical trial methods. *Phys Ther* 1995;75:93-104.

78. Harte AA, Baxter GD, Gracey JH: The efficacy of traction for back pain: A systematic review of randomized controlled trials. *Arch Phys Med Rehabil* 2003;84:1542-1553.

79. Cherkin DC, Deyo RA, Battie M, Street J, Barlow W: A comparison of physical therapy, chiropractic manipulation, and provision of an educational booklet for the treatment of patients with low back pain. *N Engl J Med* 1998;339:1021-1029.

80. Koes BW, Bouter LM, Knipschild PG, et al: The effectiveness of manual therapy, physiotherapy and continued treatment by the general practitioner for chronic nonspecific back and neck complaints: Design of a randomized clinical trial. *J Manipulative Physiol Ther* 1991;14:498-502.

81. Hsieh CY, Adams AH, Tobis J, et al: Effectiveness of four conservative treatments for subacute low back pain: A randomized clinical trial. *Spine* 2002;27:1142-1148.

82. Andersson GB, Lucente T, Davis AM, Kappler RE, Lipton JA, Leurgans S: A comparison of osteopathic spinal manipulation with standard care for patients with low back pain. *N Engl J Med* 1999;341:1426-1431.

83. Hurwitz EL, Morgenstern H, Harber P, et al: A randomized trial of medical care with and without physical therapy and chiropractic care with and without physical modalities for patients with low back pain: 6-month follow-up outcomes from the UCLA low back pain study. *Spine* 2002;27:2193-2204.

84. Bronfort G, Goldsmith CH, Nelson CF, Boline PD, Anderson AV: Trunk exercise combined with spinal manipulative or NSAID therapy for chronic low back pain: A randomized, observer-blinded clinical trial. *J Manipulative Physiol Ther* 1996;19:570-582.

85. Hemmila HM, Keinanen-Kiukaanniemi SM, Levoska S, Puska P: Long-term effectiveness of bone-setting, light exercise therapy, and physiotherapy for prolonged back pain: A randomized controlled trial. *J Manipulative Physiol Ther* 2002;25:99-104.

86. Bronfort G, Haas M, Evans RL, Bouter LM: Efficacy of spinal manipulation and mobilization for low back pain and neck pain: A systematic review and best evidence synthesis. *Spine J* 2004;4:335-356.

87. Potter NA, Rothstein JM: Intertester reliability for selected clinical tests of the sacroiliac joint. *Phys Ther* 1985;65:1671-1675.

88. Dreyfuss P, Dryer S, Griffin J, Hoffman J, Walsh N: Positive sacroiliac screening tests in asymptomatic adults. *Spine* 1994;19:1138-1143.

89. Slipman CW, Whyte WS, Ellen MI, Vresilovic EJ: Diagnosing and managing sacroiliac pain. *J Musculoskel Med* 2001;18:325-332.

90. Tullberg T, Blomberg S, Branth B, Johnsson R: Manipulation does not alter the position of the sacroiliac joint: A roentgen stereophotogrammetric analysis. *Spine* 1998;23:1124-1128.

91. Donelson R: The Mckenzie approach to evaluating and treating low back pain. *Orthop Rev* 1990;8:681-686.

92. Delitto A, Cibulka MT, Erhard RE, Bowling RW, Tenhula JA: Evidence for use of an extension-mobilization category in acute low back syndrome: A prescriptive validation pilot study. *Phys Ther* 1993;73:216-222.

93. Riddle DL, Rothstein JM: Intertester reliability of McKenzie's classifications of the syndrome types present in patients with low back pain. *Spine* 1993;18:1333-1344.

94. Saal JA: Dynamic muscular stabilization in the nonoperative treatment of lumbar pain syndromes. *Orthop Rev* 1990;19:691-700.

95. Akuthota V, Nadler SF: Core strengthening. *Arch Phys Med Rehabil* 2004;85(suppl 1):S86-S92.

96. Bigos SJ, et al: Acute Low Back Problems in Adults: Assessment and Treatment. Quick Reference Guide for Clinicians No. 14. AHCPR Publication No 95-0643. Rockville, MD, Agency for Health Care Policy and Research, U.S. Department of Health and Human Services, 1994.

97. van Tulder MW, Assendelft WJ, Koes BW, Bouter LM: Method guidelines for systematic reviews in the Cochrane

Collaboration Back Review Group for Spinal Disorders. *Spine* 1997;22:2323-2330.

98. Faas A, Chavannes AW, van Eijk JT, Gubbels JW: A randomized, placebo-controlled trial of exercise therapy in patients with acute low back pain. *Spine* 1993;18:1388-1395.

99. Stankovic R, Johnell O: Conservative treatment of acute low-back pain: A prospective randomized trial. McKenzie method of treatment versus patient education in "mini back school." *Spine* 1990;15:120-123.

100. Donchin M, Woolf O, Kaplan L, Floman Y: Secondary prevention of low-back pain: A clinical trial. *Spine* 1990;15:1317-1320.

101. Hides JA, Jull GA, Richardson CA: Long-term effects of specific stabilizing exercises for first-episode low back pain. *Spine* 2001;26:E243-E248.

102. van Tulder M, Malmivaara A, Esmail R, Koes B: Exercise therapy for low back pain: A systematic review within the framework of the Cochrane collaboration back review group. *Spine* 2000;25:2784-2796.

103. NIH Consensus Conference: Acupuncture. *JAMA* 1998;280:1518-1524.

104. Ernst E, White AR: Acupuncture for back pain: A meta-analysis of randomized controlled trials. *Arch Intern Med* 1998;158:2235-2241.

105. van Tulder MW, Cherkin DC, Berman B, Lao L, Koes BW: The effectiveness of acupuncture in the management of acute and chronic low back pain: A systematic review within the framework of the Cochrane Collaboration Back Review Group. *Spine* 1999;24:1113-1123.

106. Cherkin DC, Eisenberg D, Sherman KJ, et al: Randomized trial comparing traditional Chinese medical acupuncture, therapeutic massage, and self-care education for chronic low back pain. *Arch Intern Med* 2001;161:1081-1087.

CHAPTER 4

DIAGNOSTIC EVALUATION OF CHRONIC LOW BACK PAIN

STEVEN S. LEE, MD
ANH QUAN Q. NGUYEN, DO
DAVID FISH, MD
JEFFREY WANG, MD

Most common symptoms of chronic low back pain (LBP) have no specific anatomic diagnosis, despite clinical and radiographic testing.[1] The complex psychological, social, and economic factors in patients with chronic LBP do little to help formulate a diagnosis or a treatment plan. Advances in imaging technology, including MRI with more powerful magnets and sequence-specific imaging, have improved resolution and identification of anatomic structures without increasing the specificity of findings in patients with symptomatic back pain and in asymptomatic volunteers.[2-4] Secondary diagnostic and provocative testing has been used to help identify the "correct" source of back pain.[5,6] Many clinicians use procedures such as diskography to help make surgical decisions. However, the use of provocative testing remains controversial because false-positive results remain relatively high, and a consistently strong correlation between positive findings and surgical results has not been established.[7,8]

With judicious use of laboratory and radiographic studies, serious conditions can be distinguished from the more common degenerative changes in the lumbar spine. Any concerning signs or symptoms that could signify a more serious nonmechanical spine problem, such as malignancy or infection, are promptly identified. Imaging and further diagnostic testing can then be used to rule out these less common, but more serious, underlying conditions. Once the diagnosis is made, additional diagnostic procedures can be performed to help select the appropriate treatment plan.

Before any test is ordered, however, a systematic thorough history and physical examination are necessary. Imaging studies and further diagnostic testing are then used to corroborate physical examination findings in patients with mechanical spine conditions to confirm a suspected diagnosis. Following this sequence can lead to proper patient selection if surgical treatment is indicated and ultimately reduce the number of patients who undergo unnecessary back surgery.

TABLE 1

Differential Diagnosis of Low Back Pain

Mechanical Low Back or Leg Pain	Visceral Disease	Nonmechanical Spinal Conditions
Lumbar strain or sprain	*Pelvic organ involvement*	*Neoplasia*
Degenerative processes of the disk and facets (usually related to age)	Prostatitis	Multiple myeloma
	Endometriosis	Metastatic carcinoma
Herniated disk	Chronic pelvic inflammatory disease	Lymphoma and leukemia
Spinal stenosis		
Osteoporotic compression fracture	*Renal involvement*	*Infection*
Spondylolisthesis	Nephrolithiasis	Osteomyelitis
	Pyelonephritis	Septic diskitis
Traumatic fracture	Perinephric abscess	Paraspinous abscess
Congenital disease		Epidural abscess
Spondylolysis	Aortic aneurysm	
		Inflammatory arthritis
Internal disk disruption or discogenic back pain	*Gastrointestinal involvement*	Ankylosing spondylitis
		Psoriatic arthritis
Presumed instability	Pancreatitis	Reiter syndrome
	Cholecystitis	Inflammatory bowel disease
	Penetrating ulcer	Scheuermann's disease
		Paget's disease

(Reproduced with permission from Deyo RA, Weinstein JN: Low back pain. *N Engl J Med* 2001,344:363-370.)

HISTORY

The differential diagnosis of chronic LBP is formulated from the patient's history. The causes of LBP can be divided into three main categories: mechanical low back or leg pain (97% of patients), visceral disease (2%), and nonmechanical spine conditions (~1%).[9-11] The description of the patient's pain and perceived neurologic deficits can direct the clinician to one of these major categories[12] (Table 1).

A history of radiating leg pain with associated paresthesias can signify classic nerve root compression from a herniated disk. Straining, sneezing, coughing, or the Valsalva maneuver can exacerbate this pain. Symptoms of neurogenic claudication associated with prolonged standing or walking downhill that are relieved by sitting or assuming a hunched forward posture can indicate spinal stenosis in older patients. An inflammatory arthropathy may be suspected in younger patients with progressive back pain and morning stiffness that improve after exercise. Mild trauma with persistent back pain in a patient with osteoporosis suggests compression fractures. The sensation of spine movement or instability with changes in position can be associated with spondylolisthesis. A history of prior spine surgery can narrow the differential diagnosis, and previous surgical reports can be invaluable in guiding further treatment.

Symptoms still can remain vague and nonpecific, despite all of the above diagnoses with their classic presentations. Both symptoms and diagnoses overlap in clinical practice, in part because patients usually do not describe their symptoms in the precise medical terms clinicians use to pinpoint a diagnosis.

TABLE 2

Warning Signs of Chronic Low Back Pain

Medical Considerations	Pain Quality	Other
Cancer history	Night pain	Workers' compensation claim pending
Unexpected weight loss (>10 lb)	Progressively worsening	
Diabetes mellitus	Not improved by positional change	Active litigation
Immune deficiency		Psychiatric comorbidities
Immunosuppresion	Not improved by analgesics	
	Not improved by rest	Smoking
Advanced age		
	Change in pain character	Illicit drug use
Recent surgical procedure		
Recent infection		

Most patients have uncomplicated LBP associated with musculoskeletal sprains and strains and common degenerative changes without neurologic deficit.[1] The more serious ailments associated with back pain are found in a minority of patients.[13] The strength of the history lies in its ability to screen for medical conditions such as malignancy, infection, or nonspinal visceral diseases that can cause chronic LBP. Obtaining a complete history and conducting an adequate review of systems can reveal some of the warning signs to these more uncommon, but serious, conditions (Table 2).

A history of cancer, smoking, unexpected weight loss, and age can be associated with a malignancy in the lumbar spine. The most common malignancy in the spine is a metastatic tumor, which usually arises from a primary breast, lung, or prostate cancer. Pain is the most common presenting symptom for patients with metastatic lesions to the spine.

Progressively worsening or unremitting pain that is not relieved by rest or any changes in position may be a sign of an underlying nonmechanical spine problem. Night pain is another warning sign of a more serious condition.

A change in chronic pain, the development of saddle anesthesia, and bowel or bladder incontinence should be recognized as cauda equina syndrome. Chronic symptoms may have been present, but any new changes should be identified.

Diabetes mellitus, immune deficiency disorders, and iatrogenic immunocompromise in solid organ transplant recipients also should be noted because infections of the spine are more common in these populations than in normal, healthy populations.[14,15] Intravenous drug abuse, recent infection, or prior surgical procedures such as urologic surgery should increase suspicion for possible infectious etiology of back pain.[16-18]

Finally, some patients might have a heightened pain response or pain syndrome that can mimic the symptoms of serious spine pathology. Further physical examination and diagnostic evaluation, however, may not reveal any significant spine-related or medical condition. In this small percentage of patients, histrionic behavior or overexaggeration of pain may mask other underlying factors contributing to chronic LBP.[19,20] In these situations, various psychological, social, and economic factors need to be recognized for appropriate treatment to be administered. Results of surgical treatment are inferior when litigation or workers' compensation issues are involved.[21-23] It may be easy to discredit the patient's symptoms if these secondary gain issues are uncovered. However, a patient's report of severe, unremitting LBP necessitates further diagnostic evaluation to ensure that a spinal infection, malignancy, or visceral condition is not the real cause of the symptoms.

PHYSICAL EXAMINATION

Although many elements of the physical examination may be nonspecific, the examination complements the history in identifying significant findings that can be related to serious causes of chronic LBP. The examination should focus on and probe any of the warning signs uncovered in the initial history. Fever, tachycardia, and blood pressure changes should be noted. A general physical examination can reveal lymphadenopathy, and focused examinations can find masses in the abdominal, rectal, or pelvic regions.

The spine should be examined in patients with mechanical spine pain. Any abnormalities in sagittal and coronal alignment and range of motion should be noted. Increasing pain in forward lumbar flexion can signify disk pathology, whereas relief of back and leg pain in slight flexion may be related to spinal stenosis.[24]

The neurologic assessment includes thorough sensory, motor, and reflex testing of the spinal nerve roots innervating the lower extremities. Provocative testing, such as the straight leg test and cross straight leg test, are then performed.[25]

Problems with the hip joint, the sacroiliac joint (SIJ), and the greater trochanter can complicate identifying the source of LBP. Osteoarthritis of the hip is a common condition and can coexist with spinal pathology.[26] Careful assessment of limited and painful hip range of motion can help determine which of the two may generate the most pain. Recent reports also have implicated greater trochanteric bursitis as a source of pain that can replicate the radiating pain of problems such as spinal stenosis.[27] The SIJ is difficult to assess clinically. Although hip flexion with abduction and the external rotation test applies stress to this joint, the reproducibility and clinical utility of these tests are controversial.[12,28]

Finally, the patient's affect and physical and emotional responses to the examination can provide valuable insight into the overall pain response. Waddell's signs of nonorganic causes of LBP remain clinically useful in predicting surgical outcome.[19]

LABORATORY TESTS

Laboratory tests have limited use in the diagnostic evaluation of chronic LBP. Obtaining routine laboratory tests on every patient is unwarranted; results are neither fruitful nor cost effective in identifying a serious underlying condition in the absence of a high suspicion of nonspine-related conditions.

A complete blood count (CBC) with differential and erythrocyte sedimentation rate (ESR) can be obtained when any warning signs are identified on the history or the physical examination. The ESR can be elevated in infectious and malignant processes involving the spine. However, because ESR is a general marker of inflammation, it may have a relatively high sensitivity but poor specificity.

The CBC can identify conditions such as anemia related to a chronic disease or systemic illness. The differential may help to identify further pathology. A left shift with an increase in segmented neutrophils and bands is noted in infection. Increased lymphocytes can be noted in leukemia and other blood disorders.

With these abnormal findings, further disease-specific laboratory tests can be ordered. The type of test depends on the specific clinical history and examination findings.

PLAIN RADIOGRAPHY
Standard Views

Plain radiographs of the lumbar spine usually are the first diagnostic test ordered in the evaluation of chronic LBP. A systematic, repeatable evaluation of the radiographs will decrease the likelihood of missing subtle findings and help avoid obvious errors. This evaluation starts with identifying and confirming the correct patient identification information and noting where the right or left side markers are located.

Standard AP and lateral radiographs are useful in evaluating bony alignment and anatomy. Features such as the number of lumbar vertebrae, the presence of a sacralized distal lumbar vertebra, or other variations at the lumbosacral junction should be noted because these structures are important in preoperative planning.

The lumbar vertebrae should be counted and marked on the film, beginning with L1, to avoid confusion with future evaluation, documentation, and preoperative planning. Vertebral body and disk height also are evaluated, as is the overall quality and density of bone. Deformities, compression fractures, curvature, and spondylosis are easily seen on these views. Static spondylolisthesis also can be measured. When possible, the proximal hip joints and the sacroiliac joints should be included on the AP view. These two areas often are overlooked as a source of back pain. For inflammatory spondyloarthropathy, sacroiliitis occurs early and can be seen on radiographs. The usual stigmata of osteitis, syndesmophytosis, bony erosions, and ankylosis are evident later.

Plain radiographs are of limited value as a screening test.[29] However, they are excellent for identifying common degenerative changes, including osteophyte formation, subchondral sclerosis, and loss of intervertebral disk height, seen in much of the general population but not related to chronic LBP. Malignant lesions and spine-related infection may not be identified by plain radiographs until relatively late in the clinical course. Furthermore, soft-tissue structures that may be directly related to mechanical spine pain are not visualized on plain radiographs.

Metastatic lesions to the spine may be either lytic, blastic, or both. Although blastic lesions may be identified on radiographs earlier because of their radiodensity, approximately 50% of the trabecular bone of the vertebral body must be destroyed before a lytic lesion will be seen on radiographs.[30,31] Identification of these lesions in the posterior elements can be even more difficult because of soft-tissue shadows and bony overlap of the pedicles and laminae. Therefore, all the pedicles must be counted and any asymmetry must be noted on the AP view. The bone quality of the vertebral bodies must be compared on both views to identify any differences and any potential lesion. Lytic or blastic lesions found on plain radiographs have a 60% sensitivity and 99% specificity for cancer.[32]

Compression fractures usually are easily identified on plain radiographs. However, identifying a fracture as the source of chronic back pain can be difficult if the patient has multiple fractures or spondylosis. Radiographs cannot reveal persistent biologic activity in the bone related to healing or acuity of injury. Therefore, decisions about definitive treatment depend on findings of advanced imaging studies.

Radiographic changes in the presence of spine infec-tion occur relatively late in the disease process. In adults, infections generally are hematogenous and begin at the vertebral end plates and then extend to the adjacent structures. Loss of disk height, osteolysis, and loss of cortical margins can be seen on radiographs only after several weeks of symptoms.[33]

Special Views and Considerations

The routine use of oblique and spot lateral views is no longer recommended because neither view appears to add any further helpful clinical information.[34,35] Oblique views show the pars interarticularis in profile to identify spondylolysis but should be ordered only when clinical suspicion for this diagnosis is high.

Flexion-extension lateral views help in the evaluation of dynamic instability and may have a role in preoperative planning to determine which levels should be included in lumbar fusion. Routine use of these views is not justified unless clinically indicated or if needed for preoperative planning.[36,37]

Obtaining radiographs of the lumbar spine is not without potential risks. The amount of radiation used to penetrate the soft tissues is relatively high. The gonads, notably in women of childbearing age, are especially susceptible to the effects of repeated irradiation. Adding oblique views will expose patients to twice as much radiation as standard AP and lateral views. Radiation exposure to the gonads from standard views alone has been calculated to be equivalent to the amount of radiation exposure from a chest radiograph obtained daily for several years. [38,39]

Patient views and perceptions of the importance of plain radiographs for evaluation of chronic LBP are very strong. One study reported that patients who were inappropriately referred for radiographs tended to rate the importance of lumbar radiographs higher than patients who were appropriately referred.[40] One of the principal reasons that plain radiographs are ordered too often in the initial evaluation of LBP is patient expectations. Some patients believe that radiographs will identify the source of their back pain. Unfortunately, standard views of the lumbar spine identify problems directly related to mechanical spine pain.[41] Plain radiographs do little more than rule out the most serious underlying pathology because mild to moderate degenerative changes can be very common in both symptomatic and asymptomatic patients.

Because of the limitations of plain radiography, more

advanced imaging studies are recommended for diagnostic evaluation. Both CT and MRI provide higher sensitivity and specificity for systemic illness and degenerative conditions with neurologic compromise.

COMPUTED TOMOGRAPHY

Diagnostic CT

CT remains an important diagnostic imaging study to evaluate spinal pathology.[42] For certain indications, CT often is preferred to evaluate chronic LBP. CT uses ionizing radiation to provide excellent visualization of bony detail, as well as soft-tissue and intervertebral disk abnormalities.[43,44] These cross-sectional images also can be reformatted in the sagittal and coronal planes and as three-dimensional models to improve visualization of complex spinal anatomy. In most instances, however, it is reserved as a secondary choice.[3] MRI has largely replaced CT for initial evaluation of chronic LBP because of its excellent ability to visualize soft tissue and maintain adequate bony detail. CT, however, remains quite useful in patients for whom MRI is contraindicated. CT has been reported to have similar sensitivity and specificity to MRI in detecting herniated disks.[45,46]

Because CT provides excellent visualization of bony anatomy, central and foraminal stenosis resulting from osteophytes or other bony abnormalities is easily seen.[47] This allows accurate assessment of the location and levels of stenosis, which can then be correlated with anatomic and physical examination findings.

Degenerative changes of the facet joint are better visualized with CT than with MRI.[48,49] Facet joints have been implicated as a source of LBP in the absence of other anatomic abnormalities. Degenerative disease most commonly occurs at L4-5 and L5-S1 because this area of the lumbar spine bears the most weight. Cartilage destruction leads to peripheral osteophytes, subchondral cysts, and joint hypertrophy.

If vertebroplasty or kyphoplasty is being considered as treatment of osteoporotic compression fractures, CT is helpful to confirm the fracture pattern. Compression fractures must be differentiated from burst fractures, and any fracture lines extending through the end plate should be noted. Identifying the fracture pattern and the extent of the fracture is important so that cement does not extrude out of the vertebral body and into the surrounding soft tissues and the spinal canal.

Postoperative CT

Postoperatively, CT has certain advantages over MRI because of the improved bone visualization. In some situations, patients with chronic LBP may have had prior spine surgery, with or without instrumentation. The best images are seen in patients without instrumentation because there is no metal artifact. Bone resection from prior laminotomy or laminectomy can be seen and is helpful in considering revision surgery. The position of the pedicle screws can be visualized to determine if a violation through the bony cortex may be causing symptoms related to nerve root irritation. Finally, the quality of a bony fusion mass can be evaluated.

CT Myelography

CT myelography combines bony detail with visualization of neural elements. Unfortunately, myelography is reported to be unpleasant and painful for patients.[50] It is a poor option for initial evaluation because MRI can visualize the spinal cord and nerves well; thus, myelography should be reserved for patients in whom MRI is contraindicated. Because the radiopaque dye used in CT myelography cannot pass through a complete block, anatomy beyond a level of stenosis may not be visualized. There also are rare instances of rapid neurologic deterioration with the introduction of increased volume.[51]

MAGNETIC RESONANCE IMAGING

MRI has become the initial diagnostic imaging study of choice after plain radiography for the evaluation of chronic LBP. MRI has several advantages over CT for imaging of the spine; it does not require the use of ionizing radiation; it provides better distinction between different types of soft tissues; and it offers improved visualization of any changes or abnormalities in the bone marrow of the vertebral bodies and the elements within the spinal canal.

The imaging sequences (ie, T1 weighted and T2 weighted) capitalize on the differences in energy release of the protons in various soft tissues in response to the strong magnetic field. Stronger magnetic fields improve image quality. Any changes in bone marrow, specifically neoplasm, infection, reactive edema, and degenerative changes, are best detected by T1-weighted images. T2-

weighted images best visualize the spinal cord, nerve roots, canal dimensions, and edema.

The use of gadolinium as a contrast medium is not recommended in the routine initial evaluation of the spine. Data on its value in identifying nerve root enhancement are not consistent.[52,53] In patients who have not had prior spine surgery, use of contrast is not recommended. In certain clinical situations, however, gadolinium can help in the identification and diagnosis of a particular disease process. Patients who have had prior spine surgery and patients believed to have infectious or malignant processes involving the spine would benefit from the addition of contrast because these agents enhance areas of abnormality.

Disk Pathology

Degenerative disk disease is characterized by a loss in disk height and decreased signal intensity on T2-weighted images. This classic appearance has been termed the "black disk" and is the result of disk dehydration and loss of integrity of the collagen infrastructure. In severe disk degeneration, the collapse of the intervertebral space, and an occasional "vacuum" disk phenomenon can occur. The collapsed disk can contain nitrogen gas that is seen on radiographs, CT, and MRI.[54,55] Vertebral end-plate changes associated with disk degeneration also have been described.

Modic and associates[56] described three types of changes based on differences in T1 and T2 signal intensity. Type I changes represent vascularized marrow with low T1 signal intensity and high T2 signal intensity. This stage is believed to be inflammatory, with increased symptoms and functional disability. Type II changes represent chronic degenerative disease that occurs after the initial inflammatory stage as a natural progression of disk degeneration. After lumbar fusion to stabilize the spine, type II changes have been reported to appear after 6 months. Correcting the mechanical instability was believed to accelerate the changes in end-plate progression[57] that are associated with fatty marrow changes with high signal on T1-weighted images and iso- or hyperintense signal on T2-weighted images. Type III changes are characterized by low signal on both T1- and T2-weighted images and represent dense bone without marrow. Some authors correlate these Modic changes with symptoms of back pain; however, the utility of this classification remains

controversial because other authors report poor correlation with MRI end-plate changes and concordant diskography findings.[58,59]

Disk herniation is believed to contribute to chronic back pain, and many authors have described this condition. Brant-Zawadzki and Jensen[60] described a nomenclature system based on the appearance of disk morphology on MRI. (1) A normal disk does not extend beyond the posterior vertebral body. (2) A disk bulge extends diffusely beyond the vertebral body margin in all directions. (3) A disk protrusion is a focal, broad-based extension of the disk into the canal, with the base of the protrusion broader than the extent of protrusion, and an associated displacement of disk material through a defect in the inner annular fibers with some outer annular fibers remaining intact. (4) Finally, a disk extrusion is a focal extension of disk material into the spinal canal, with the base of the extrusion narrower than the extent of extrusion. Extrusion differs from protrusion in that the former involves a defect in which disk material extrudes through both inner and outer annular fibers. Subligamentous extrusions are disk material that remains anterior to the posterior longitudinal ligament, and free or sequestered disk fragments are disk material that is no longer in continuity with the native disk. These free fragments can migrate caudal or cephalad to the level of their original disk and cause symptoms based on their final location.

Disk herniation is seen well on T2-weighted images because the disk material displaces the high-signal cerebrospinal fluid. The position of posterolateral and lateral disk herniations can be further localized on T1-weighted images because the disk displaces the high signal of fat in the epidural space and foramen.

The tear in the anulus fibers associated with disk herniations seen on MRI has been termed the high-intensity zone (HIZ). A focal high-intensity signal on T2-weighted images in the posterior anulus is believed to represent the defect. The clinical importance of this radiographic finding remains controversial.[6] Authors have reported findings ranging from high correlation to no correlation of the presence of this HIZ and concordant diskography findings.[58,61-63]

The major difficulty in implicating degenerative disk disease and disk herniations as an obvious cause of chronic LBP is the prevalence of these findings in a significant proportion of asymptomatic people. HIZs can be found in as many as 38% of a study group.[29,61] Disk herniations ranging from bulges to protrusions are present in roughly 30% to 50% of an asymptomatic study group, but extrusions are present in only 1%.[4,64] Although these reports may seem discouraging, they must be interpreted in the context of patient age. The more significant findings of disk extrusion, end-plate changes, and nerve compression are much less common in patients younger than age 50 years and may directly correlate with LBP in that group.[64,65]

Stenosis

Central, lateral recess, and foraminal stenosis in the lumbar spine may be related to chronic LBP. Osteophytes, facet joint arthropathy, bulging disks, and thickened ligamentum flavum can be associated with stenosis,[66] which is seen on MRI by compression or distortion of the thecal sac or loss of visualization of the epidural fat surrounding the neural structures.

Central stenosis is classified as mild, moderate, or severe. Radiologists have quantified stenosis to be less than 1.5 cm² in total area or less than 11.5 mm in AP diameter.[67,68] Using these parameters, however, is more difficult in clinical practice.

Lateral recess stenosis, defined as the loss of normal space between the anterior border of the superior articular facet and the posterior border of the vertebral body, often can be seen in conjunction with central stenosis. The spinal nerve leaves the central canal through the lateral recess where osteophytes, facet joint hypertrophy, and disk herniation or bulges can compress the nerve root. On MRI, facet joint arthropathy usually is identified by fluid in the joint, the presence of facet cysts, and the abnormal morphology of the joint itself.

Foraminal stenosis affects the exiting nerve root and is seen best on the sagittal images. Normally, the surrounding epidural fat produces a bright signal, with the T1-weighted images highlighting the nerve root[69] (Figure 1). This "halo" around the nerve disappears with foraminal stenosis.

No clear consensus has been reached on the exact determination of what defines mild versus severe stenosis. In fact, only a fair level of agreement exists among observers in describing the amount of stenosis at the lateral recess or foramen. Only the assessment of the degree of central stenosis is consistent among observers.[70]

FIGURE 1

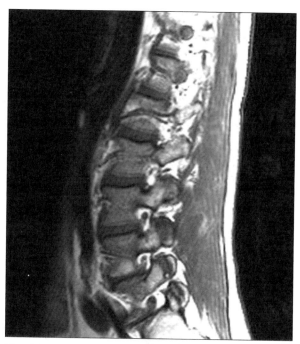

T1-weighted sagittal image of a normal neural foramina. Note the normal "halo" surrounding the nerve root as it exits the foramina.

Functional MRI

The use of functional MRI to evaluate LBP has been of some interest. With the advent of new open MRI machines, patients can be placed in upright and seated positions rather than in the standard supine position. Images also can be taken in flexion and extension to simulate physiologic conditions.[71,72] In certain patients these studies may demonstrate clinically relevant neural compromise, foraminal stenosis, or disk pathology not seen with the typical supine, non–weight-bearing images. Whether these findings improve treatment outcomes has not yet been demonstrated.

Infection

The identification of a spine infection can be difficult without a high degree of suspicion. Because plain radiographic changes at the vertebral end plate may not be identified until later in the disease process, MRI has become the imaging study of choice to detect infectious processes in the spine.[33,73,74] As mentioned earlier, the use of contrast enhancement helps with diagnosis.

The most specific sign of infection on MRI is the destruction of the vertebral end plate and edema within the vertebral bodies adjacent to the involved disk. The involved disk and the adjacent vertebrae can be identified by high signal intensity in the T2-weighted images. Disk space narrowing or even the complete destruction of the disk can be seen in chronic osteomyelitis or diskitis.

Both malignancy and infection can manifest with osteolysis and destruction of the vertebral body. Note, however, that tumors almost never involve the disk space, whereas infection results in destruction of the disk.

Malignancy

MRI is more sensitive in detecting metastatic disease and primary malignant spine tumors than plain radiography, bone scan, and CT.[75,76] A diagnosis of a pathologic process is inferred from the patient's history as well as the indirect signs on the image. The T1-weighted images should be closely evaluated to detect malignant process in the vertebral body. Normal marrow has a high T1 signal intensity because of the high fat content; abnormal conditions are seen as areas of low T1 signal areas in the body.[77] Involvement of the posterior spinal elements can be well localized with MRI, and soft-tissue extension of the tumor is also seen. These images are helpful in preoperative planning.

T2-weighed images are less helpful than the T1-weighted images because malignant processes can have low, high, or the same signal intensity as the surrounding normal bone. Diseases such as myeloma, lymphoma, or leukemia that involve the entire vertebral body are seen as diffuse low T1 signal throughout the bone. More focal involvement of metastases is contrasted by focal low signal adjacent to the normal, high marrow signal on the T1-weighted images.

Pathologic fractures may be difficult to diagnose in patients with osteoporosis.[78] In the first 6 months after fracture, both benign and malignant fractures can have high T2 signal intensity because of the inflammation and increased water content, and both are dark on T1-weighted images. Diffusion-weighted MRI can distinguish pathologic from benign compression fractures.[79] Suspicious lesions at other vertebral bodies, abnormal soft-tissue extension, cortical destruction, and involvement of the posterior elements can influence the differential diagnosis toward a metastatic process.

BONE SCAN

Bone scans detect metabolically active bone. A triple-phase bone scan adds dynamic blood flow and blood pool images to the standard delayed image, thereby helping to discern hyperemia or inflammation to diagnose infection or osteomyelitis.

Bone scans currently are used in the diagnosis of active infection, metastases, and fractures. The bone scan is a fairly sensitive test for detection of both cancer and infection because these processes will be active on the bone scan; however, its specificity is only moderate.[80,81] Metastases from primary lung, breast, and prostate cancers usually have an osteoblastic response and thus are positive on bone scan, but false-negative results can arise from tumors that are slow growing or do not have a typical osteoblastic response.

Bone scans are best used to determine the acuity of a compression fracture found on plain radiographs. Acute or biologically active fractures in the midst of multiple old fractures should appear on the bone scan and help identify proper levels for treatment.[82]

The most appropriate use of a bone scan appears to be the confirmation or exclusion of a suspected diagnosis. Bone scans may be most effective in excluding tumor, infection, or occult fracture. CT and MRI, however, have largely replaced bone scans because of their higher sensitivity and specificity and because they provide more anatomic information that may affect future treatment. These advanced imaging tests also should be used to confirm a diagnosis rather than to identify abnormalities.

SECONDARY DIAGNOSTIC PROCEDURES

The history and examination findings sometimes do not correlate well with the imaging studies.[83] Not infrequently only common degenerative changes are seen on MRI, with no specific finding to explain LBP. The sources of LBP are numerous, including annular tears, nerve root impingement, facet arthropathy, or SIJ problems among others. Which of these potential pain generators, then, is responsible for generating the pain?

Because physical examination findings and radiographic images fail to definitively identify the cause of LBP, other diagnostic procedures are used, specifically fluoroscopically guided diagnostic and therapeutic spinal interventions. These can help with diagnosis and treatment planning, but neither are infallible and are used best in conjunction with the history, physical examination, and electrodiagnostic studies. Diagnostic blocks can be especially helpful in patients whose physical examination and imaging studies are essentially normal. The value of these diagnostic procedures has been questioned in the literature; nevertheless, they remain an invaluable tool to narrow the differential diagnosis of chronic LBP. When used appropriately, these tests can help pinpoint the appropriate treatment and ultimately may improve patient outcomes.

Electromyography

The needle electromyography (EMG) is an electrophysiologic study that is most often used to evaluate the acuity and severity of cervical or lumbar radiculopathy, although it can for other conditions such as myopathy, anterior horn cell disease, and neuromuscular transmission defects. A needle electrode is placed into limb and paraspinal muscles to evaluate the motor unit in a two-stage process. The first stage assesses the muscle and motor units while at rest for spontaneous activity, indications of membrane instability, axonal injury, or denervation. The second stage assesses the muscles during mild, moderate, and full-effort contractions for motor unit amplitude, duration, and phasicity. These parameters can help identify motor unit drop out, signs of reinnervation, and chronicity. The diagnosis of radiculopathy is made if abnormal electrophysiologic findings occur in two separate muscles sharing the same nerve root but innervated by different peripheral nerves.

Needle EMG has been shown to correlate well with MRI findings. Nardin and associates[84] reported a 60% correlation between abnormal EMG findings and MRI findings in patients designated as having definite radiculopathy (ie, clear radicular symptoms, abnormal physical examination findings, and clinical history compatible with radiculopathy). The authors also reported that MRI tended to show equally high rates of imaging abnormalities in patients defined as having definite and those with only possible radiculopathy (60% and 57%, respectively), unlike EMG, which was abnormal in 72% and 29% of patients, respectively. These findings suggest a lack of specificity in MRI compared with EMG in the diagnosis of radiculopathy. This lack of specificity has

been supported by other authors who have studied and reported significant spine MRI abnormalities in asymptomatic individuals.[4,64]

Tsao and associates[85] reported that when EMG and MRI or CT findings agreed on a level of pathology, there was a strong correlation with surgical findings. Their study evaluated 45 patients with a preoperative diagnosis of unilateral lumbosacral radiculopathy with sustained denervation potentials and abnormal MRI or CT imaging. All 45 patients meeting the inclusion criteria had a surgically confirmed "visibly distorted, compromised or otherwise compressed single nerve root."

Needle EMG is clearly helpful in determining if a radiculopathy is present. However, electrophysiologic changes generally are not present before 7 to 10 days after nerve injury, and early testing may be normal. In addition, needle EMG is better at "ruling in" a diagnosis of radiculopathy than ruling it out because a lack of abnormalities simply may be a function of sampling an area where there were no denervation changes.

Diskography

Discogenic back pain refers to pain in the lumbar spine without evidence of disk herniation or nerve root impingement. The pain is believed to result from disruption of the internal annular fibers, which have free nerve endings, and can radiate into the lower extremities. Diskography is a purely diagnostic tool that is used most often to determine if the pain can be attributed to a problem with the disk itself. Results are used to determine if surgical treatment such as a spinal fusion is an option. With diskography, a nonirritating contrast agent is injected to distend the disk, activating pain nociceptors and ultimately reproducing the patient's pain. Injection of a normal disk should be pain free.

Early studies by Holt[86] revealed a high false-positive rate of pain production when diskography was performed in an asymptomatic volunteer prison population. Walsh and associates,[87] in a limited study of 10 men with no history of LBP and a control group of seven men with a 6-month history of LBP, performed diskography on a total of 30 disks while videotaping the patients to assess pain-related behaviors. In this study, a positive diskogram showed abnormal imaging and produced substantial pain on testing. The authors reported a 0% false-positive rate.

Carragee and associates[88] performed a similar study

in which 20 patients with no history of LBP but with a history of cervical fusion or diskectomy (10 pain free, 10 with chronic neck/arm pain) and six with somatization disorders based on *Diagnostic and Statistical Manual of Mental Disorders*, ed 4, (DSM IV) criteria underwent lumbar diskography. Of these patients, 10% of the patients who were pain free, 40% who had had surgical failures, and 83% of the patients with somatization disorders had a significant positive pain response and related behaviors. These results suggest that patients with abnormal psychometric testing or chronic pain are much more likely to report painful disk injections.

In a different study, these authors[89] evaluated the issue of concordancy when they illustrated the poor reliability of patient reports on concordant pain. Diskography was performed in eight patients with normal psychometric testing and no history of LBP, despite findings of degenerative disk disease or annular tears on imaging studies. All of these patients had undergone iliac crest bone grafting for non–spine-related procedures. On injection, seven of the 24 disks tested produced similar and two had exact reproduction of gluteal pain or LBP since iliac grafting. These findings question whether concordant pain reported during diskography really represented pain emanating from the spine. Because all of the patients had either disk degeneration or tears, their reports of pain over the iliac crest area certainly could be from a pathologic disk referring pain to the same postoperative area.

Derby and associates[90] studied the use of manometric diskography with specific criteria for a positive diskogram. They defined a positive diskogram as one that reproduces concordant pain (ie, described as at least 6 of 10 on a numeric rating scale), with less than 50 psi of intradiskal pressure with injection and less than 3.5 mL of injected volume. In their study of 16 patients (7 asymptomatic, 6 occasional LBP, 3 frequent LBP), careful use of manometric-guided diskography and these criteria resulted in "no false positives for the diagnosis of discogenic LBP." Table 3 lists the indications for diskography based on the most recent position statement by the North American Spine Society.[91]

The technique of diskography is critical. A nonionic, nonirritating contrast dye is injected into the suspected disk and a control disk while simultaneously asking the patient to report whether the pain with injection is similar, dissimilar, or exactly the same as his or her usual

TABLE 3
North American Spine Society Indications for Diskography
1. Further evaluation of demonstrably abnormal disks to help assess the extent of abnormality or to correlate the abnormality with the clinical symptoms, which may include recurrent pain from a previously surgically treated disk and lateral disk herniations.
2. Assessment of patients with persistent, severe symptoms in whom other diagnostic tests have failed to clearly confirm a suspected disk as the source of pain.
3. Assessment of patients who have not responded to surgical interventions to identify painful pseudarthrosis or a symptomatic disk in a posteriorly fused segment and to help evaluate possible recurrent disk herniation.
4. Assessment of disks before fusion to identify symptomatic disks within the proposed fusion segment and to determine if disks adjacent to this segment are normal.
5. Assessment of candidates for minimally invasive surgical intervention to confirm a contained disk herniation or to investigate the dye distribution pattern before chemonucleolysis or percutaneous procedures.

pain. The most recent position statement by the North American Spine Society recommends recording the volume of contrast, the pain response with the location of pain, and the pattern of dye seen in addition to concordancy. In a normal disk, the contrast should be well centered with smooth margins outlined. Contrast that goes out of the nuclear zone indicates disruption of the annular fibers (Figure 2).

Diskography is frequently ordered to identify the levels involved in generating pain so that definitive treatment such as lumbar fusion can be planned.

However, the literature is mixed on the ability of diskography to predict surgical outcomes.

Smith and associates[92] retrospectively reviewed the records of 25 patients who did not have surgery despite a positive diskogram. These patients had at least 6 months of nonradicular LBP that failed to respond to physical therapy. Inclusion criteria consisted of normal radiographs and a diskogram that showed concordant pain and abnormal disk appearance. Patients elected not to have surgery because of fear of complications (12), insurance denial (8), family or acquaintance with poor outcome (3), and choice of lifestyle changes (2). Results at follow-up (mean, 4.9 years) showed that symptoms improved in 68% of patients, worsened in 24%, and were unchanged in 8%. Of the patients with worse pain, 66.7% had a history of psychiatric illness, which may confound the reports of pain. This study also was limited by small sample size, its retrospective nature, and recall bias, but the results do suggest that up to two thirds of patients with nonradicular pain and a positive diskogram may improve without surgery.

Colhoun and associates[93] reported that 88% of patients with a positive diskogram had a successful outcome after fusion, whereas only 52% of those who did not have a positive diskogram had a similar outcome. In a more recent study, Madan and associates[94] evaluated 73 patients who underwent posterior lumbar interbody fusion and posterior spinal arthrodesis. Of these, 41 patients had circumferential arthrodesis but no preoperative diskogram and 32 had preoperative diskograms (with partially or wholly reproduced pain with diskography). Both groups had satisfactory outcomes (75.6% without diskography, 81.2% with diskography) without a statistically significant difference between the two groups.

Derby and associates[90] measured disk pressures in an effort to provide more objective standards for use of diskography by measuring disk pressures. In a limited sample of patients with chemically sensitive disks (immediate onset of familiar pain, less than 1 mL of contrast at less than 15 psi above opening pressures, and significant pain [greater than 6 of 10 on a visual pain scale]), the results of interbody combined fusion (89%) were better than in posterior intertransverse fusion alone (20%).

Based on the available literature, the benefit and

FIGURE 2

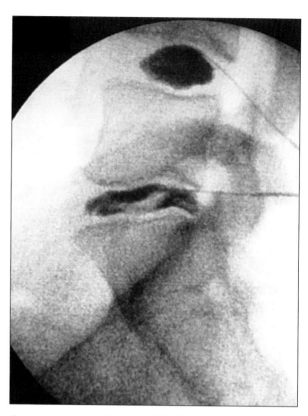

Fluoroscopic view of diskography. Note the normal disk at L4-5 with well-contained contrast material and the abnormal disk at L5-S1 with abnormal contrast distribution.

even the validity of results from diskography are still unclear. Diskography should not be used as the sole test to make a diagnosis; it should be used in conjunction with the history, physical examination findings, and imaging studies to rule out other sources of pain before it is assumed that the disk is the source of pain. Furthermore, results of diskography must be interpreted in light of the quality of the diskographer, the patient's responses, and confounding psychosocial factors.

FACET JOINT INJECTION

The facet joints generally are acknowledged as a source of LBP, with prevalence debated in the literature. Based on response to injections, the prevalence has been reported to range between 15% and 40%,[95-97] and it is variable, depending on patient selection criteria and methodology for diagnosis such as single- versus double-block injection. The facet joints consist of the inferior articular process of the cephalad vertebra paired with the superior articular process of the vertebra below. These joints are innervated at the affected level and the level above by the medial branch of the dorsal ramus, and thus have nociceptive capabilities. Goldthwaith[98] implicated the facet joints as possible sources of LBP in 1911. In 1976, Mooney and Robertson[95] reported that injecting normal saline solution into the facet joints of normal volunteers induced LBP as well as radiation of pain, confirming the joint's ability to produce pain.

The diagnosis of facet syndrome by physical examination or radiographic evidence is also controversial. Many clinicians believe that tests such as extension and rotation will stress facet joints and should reproduce facet pain. Helbig and Lee[96] attempted to create a 100-point system by which pain symptoms, imaging findings, and physical examination tests could be weighted toward the diagnosis. They reported that patients who scored higher than 60 of 100 had a "100% prolonged response." Unfortunately, patients with scores of only 40 of 100 also responded to facet joint block (FJB). In their study, pain with extension-rotation merited 30 points alone.

Revel and associates,[97] studying seven different clinical variables with the goal of identifying criteria that would predict positive response to FJB and thus the presence of facet-mediated pain, reported that patients with pain on hyperextension and extension-rotation tended not to respond to FJB. Schwarzer and associates,[99] investigating whether clinical features could determine facet-mediated pain, agreed that no "combination of historic or examination features could be used to predict pain of zygapophyseal joint origin." They believed patients with central lumbar pain were unlikely to respond to FJBs.

Imaging studies also are not useful in the diagnosis of facet-mediated pain. In a study with a controlled double injection in 63 patients, Schwarzer and associates[100] reported that CT could not differentiate patients who responded to FJB from those who did not based on the degree of osteoarthritis seen in the facet joints. Because no clear clinical or radiographic modality can be used to identify facet joints as the cause of LBP, diagnostic

injections have been the modality of choice.

The indications for performing facet joint injections are based on the International Spinal Injection Society (ISIS) 1997 guidelines for performance of spinal procedures:[101] "Lumbar zygapophyseal joint blocks may be performed in patients with low back pain for which no cause is otherwise evident and whose pain pattern resembles that evoked in normal volunteers upon stimulation of their zygapophyseal joints."

Initial studies by Mooney and Robertson[95] showed that saline solution introduced to lumbar zygapophyseal joints in normal subjects could reproduce pain into the leg, low back, groin, and greater trochanter, among other areas. More recently, Fukui and associates[102] studied facet referral pain patterns based on joint distention and medial branch electrical stimulation. They reported that the use of pain maps to identify the involved facet joint was not clinically useful because of the significant overlap of pain referral patterns.

Two procedures performed under sterile technique with fluoroscopic guidance are commonly used to aid in diagnosis of facet-mediated pain. In intra-articular facet joint injection, needles are placed into the affected joint, and contrast medium is injected to confirm proper placement. A dumbbell-shaped longitudinal slit will appear with sufficient contrast (Figure 3). In dorsal ramus medial branch block, needles are directed toward the eye of the Scottie dog; once at the neck, local anesthetic can be injected.

ISIS[101] currently recommends that patients who respond to the initial set of injections, whether to the facet joint or the medial branch, undergo a second confirmatory injection. The second injection should be done with a different anesthetic that has either a longer or shorter duration of activity than the one used in the first block. According to ISIS, a positive response occurs when the patient's pain relief from the second block correlates with the known duration of activity of the second anesthetic.

Schwarzer and associates[99] reported a large number of false-positive responses to lumbar facet joint injections. Of 47 patients who responded with definite or complete relief from initial screening lignocaine injections, only 15% responded to a second controlled confirmatory block. They reported a 38% false-positive rate for blind injections. High false-positive rates also have been reported by others.[97,103] If patients report sufficient

FIGURE 3

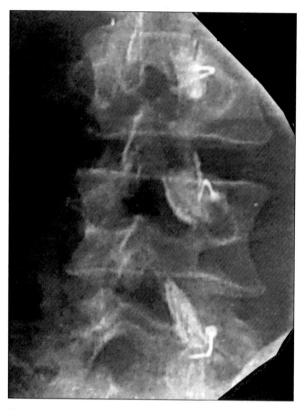

Fluoroscopic view of intra-articular facet injections.

pain relief and desire further treatment, radiofrequency (RF) ablation can be considered.

RF ablation is a procedure in which an RF electrode is guided to the superior edge of the transverse process of the involved medial branch. The electrode is evaluated radiographically to ensure that the orientation is parallel to the estimated course of the medial branch nerve, which is then stimulated to further ensure proper placement of the RF electrode. Subsequently, the electrode is heated with the goal of thermal coagulation of the medial branch nerve. If the joint is the source of the pain, coagulation and destruction of the nerve should eliminate the pain.

Dreyfuss and associates[104] performed RF ablation followed by EMG to detect denervation changes in a group of patients whose diagnosis of facet-mediated pain was based on a double block protocol. Sixty percent of the patients reported at least a 90% reduction of pain, and

87% reported at least 60% pain relief for about 12 months. In addition, the authors believed that radiographic confirmation of proper placement of the electrode was sufficient and that electrical stimulation of the nerve to verify placement was unnecessary.

Positive responses to FJB for chronic LBP have led to lumbar arthrodesis. Data are mixed regarding the ability of response to FJB to predict surgical outcomes. Esses and Moro[105] retrospectively reviewed the records of 296 patients who had FJBs done as part of a workup for LBP. Some of the 82 who had single or multiple level lumbar fusion also had had previous laminectomy, diskectomy, or fusions at other levels. The authors concluded there was no statistically significant correlation between the results of FJB and the subsequent response to surgery. Limitations of this study include recall bias; moreover, patients with reported positive FJB apparently had a single injection, rather than double controlled injections. The significant rate of reported false-positive results in single uncontrolled injections indicates that a significant proportion of the treated patients may not have had facet joint pain; thus, the study does not evaluate the response of facet joint pain to arthrodesis.

SACROILIAC JOINT INJECTION

The SIJ is a possible cause of LBP, but it is not normally considered in the differential diagnosis before the facet joints or the disks. The lack of a clear clinical history to suggest the diagnosis also is a factor, although numerous clinical examination findings and provocative procedures are thought to be diagnostic.

The International Association for the Study of Pain[106] defines SIJ pain as "spinal pain stemming from the sacroiliac joint." The diagnostic criteria for SIJ pain are as follows: (1) pain in the region of the SIJ; (2) pain that is reproduced by stressing the SIJ using clinical tests selective for the joint; or (3) pain completely relieved by selectively infiltrating the putatively symptomatic joint with local anesthetic.

Fortin and associates[107] injected contrast medium into the SIJ under fluoroscopy in a small group of healthy volunteers (Figure 4), which resulted in pain in the posterior iliac spine that radiated to the gluteus in a 3- × 10-cm vertical distribution. The authors recorded this "map" to determine if it could help distinguish patients with SIJ pain from patients with pain of another

FIGURE 4

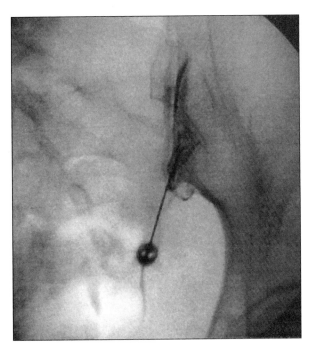

Fluoroscopic view of a successful intra-articular SIJ injection.

origin. Two clinicians independently evaluated self-reported pain diagrams from 54 patients and agreed that the diagrams of 16 patients suggested SIJ pain. All 16 patients had provocative positive contrast injections but a variable response to instilled bupivicaine, making the validity of the diagnosis using this method questionable. Only two patients reported complete pain relief, and 10 had "at least 50%" relief following injection. The response to contrast distention may be referred pain from a normally asymptomatic joint into an area that was already painful, but not an SIJ etiology, which may explain the lack of more significant relief with bupivicaine injection.

Maigne and associates[108] attempted to confirm the presence of an SIJ syndrome, as well as determine its prevalence. They evaluated 54 patients with unilateral LBP and tenderness over the SIJ, with or without pain radiation. Patients were given a screening injection with lidocaine and then a controlled injection with bupivicaine. Seven provocative tests for SIJ pain were done before and after the first injection. Based on patient response to the controlled block, the authors reported SIJ pain in 18.5% of the patients, but the relationship between provocative clinical testing and the response to the injection was not statistically significant.

The lack of provocative testing to diagnose SIJ pain also was reported by Dreyfuss and associates.[109] They assessed both seated and standing flexion and performed Gillet tests on a group of asymptomatic individuals. A total of 20% of their subjects had positive SIJ screening tests.

Schwarzer and associates[110] used SIJ injections to evaluate 43 patients with pain centered below L5-S1. All patients received a double block FJB protocol in an effort to identify those more likely to have false-positive results. Thirteen patients reported reproduction of their pain with injection of contrast agent and "definite and gratifying relief" after anesthetic instillation. No clinical feature identified patients with SIJ pain with statistical significance; however, the authors reported a statistically significant relationship between referred groin pain patterns and response to SIJ blocks. They also reported that sacral sulcus tenderness was the most sensitive test, and tenderness at the posterior superior iliac spine had the best predictive value but not to statistical significance. The testing done in this study reproduced pain but did not correlate with response to anesthetic injection. Overall, the study was well done but could have been strengthened if controlled blocks were injected in the SIJ rather than in the facet joints. A placebo response to an SIJ injection could not be ruled out, despite lack of placebo response in the facet joints.

The SIJ clearly can cause LBP, even though its prevalence is not as clear because reports in the literature vary widely. Physical examination and provocative testing, both commonly used in clinical practice, are not reliable means to make the diagnosis. Thus, use of the diagnostic injection protocol generally has been accepted as the gold standard for diagnostic evaluation.

No clear clinical guidelines exist for the use of SIJ blocks for evaluation, other than perhaps clinical suspicion and ruling out other sources of LBP. Chou and associates[111] recently evaluated 54 patients believed to have SIJ syndrome based on positive diagnostic block and subsequent therapeutic injections of betamethasone and lidocaine. The authors reported that 44% of the patients had a history of some type of trauma (eg, motor vehicle accident, fall, fracture, or postpartum), 35% had a spontaneous or idiopathic onset, and 21% had a cumulative injury (eg, lifting, running, crew training, hip extension injury). Fortin[112] also suggested these as inciting etiologies.

Physical examination with provocative testing has been an inadequate means of confirming SIJ pain, failing to withstand clinical studies of validity. Tests commonly used to confirm the diagnosis, specifically Gaenslen's, Patrick's, Yeoman's, and Gillet's tests, have not proved to be of diagnostic value.[109,113] Dreyfuss and associates[113] reported significant overlap in pain diagrams of patients who did and did not respond to SIJ blocks; however, only two patients diagnosed with SIJ-mediated pain described pain above L5, unlike patients without block-confirmed SIJ pain. This finding was not statistically significant but was suggestive.

Slipman and associates[114] evaluated the response of patients with SIJ syndrome to therapeutic injections of corticosteroid. Inclusion criteria consisted of pain over the sacral sulcus with at least three sacral provocative positive tests (eg, Patrick's, Gaenslen's, Yeoman's, and shear test) and failure of nonsurgical treatment. Patients who reported 80% pain relief with an initial injection of 2% lidocaine received a subsequent SIJ block with betamethasone and 2% lidocaine. Patients who reported more than 90% relief from the second injection, but described the relief as "progressive," received a third corticosteroid injection. Patients were followed an average of nearly 2 years. The authors found statistically significant improvement in Oswestry scores, as well as Visual Analog Pain Scale scores at the time of follow-up. Unfortunately, the study was confounded by the fact that patients had physical therapy. It is unclear what role therapy had in initial and sustained improvement of symptoms because the study data did not address this factor. The authors also pointed out that they lacked a control group and used only one diagnostic block before giving patients a therapeutic injection.

Ferrante and associates[115] recently reported the use of RF denervation and neurotomy in patients with SIJ syndrome. Initial diagnostic injections consisted of bupivicaine and betamethasone. Patients who reported more than 50% pain relief from the initial injection were offered RF denervation, in which they were given bupivacaine and betamethasone again prior to RF. The authors reported that of the 33 patients, 12 had at least 50% decrease in vascular autonomic signal for an average of 12 ± 1.2 months. This study is good but fails to control for false-positive responses to the initial bupivacaine and betamethasone injection by using a second control injection. Furthermore, the use of physical examinations to confirm a diagnosis of SIJ syndrome has been shown to be of limited benefit. Thus, the conclusions of this study would have been stronger had the patient received a double block control injection prior to RF denervation.

SUMMARY

Identifying the causes of chronic LBP is very complex because of the many different potential sources. The patient history, physical examination, and imaging studies may not lead to a clear diagnosis. However, these evaluations may be able to rule out serious nonmechanical causes of chronic pain such as spinal infection or cancer. When initial evaluations are not conclusive, secondary spinal diagnostic tests such as differential injections and diskography can be used to help pinpoint the diagnosis. These tools may help lead to stronger correlations between results of diagnostic procedures and surgical outcomes. Ultimately, the goals of diagnostic evaluation are improved surgical outcomes and patient satisfaction in the treatment of this complex disease.

REFERENCES

1. White AA III, Gordon SL: Synopsis: Workshop on idiopathic low-back pain. *Spine* 1982;7:141-149.

2. Boden SD, Wiesel SW: Lumbar spine imaging: Role in clinical decision making. *J Am Acad Orthop Surg* 1996;4:238-248.

3. Boden SD: The use of radiographic imaging studies in the evaluation of patients who have degenerative disorders of the lumbar spine. *J Bone Joint Surg Am* 1996;78:114-124.

4. Jensen MC, Brant-Zawadzki MN, Obuchowski N, Modic MT, Malkasian D, Ross JS: Magnetic resonance imaging of the lumbar spine in people without back pain. *N Engl J Med* 1994;331:69-73.

5. Milette PC, Fontaine S, Lepanto L, Cardinal E, Breton G: Differentiating lumbar disc protrusions, disc bulges, and discs with normal contour but abnormal signal intensity: Magnetic resonance imaging with discographic correlations. *Spine* 1999;24:44-53.

6. Smith BM, Hurwitz EL, Solsberg D, et al: Interobserver reliability of detecting lumbar intervertebral disc high-

intensity zone on magnetic resonance imaging and association of high-intensity zone with pain and anular disruption. *Spine* 1998;23:2074-2080.

7. Boas RA: Nerve blocks in the diagnosis of low back pain. *Neurosurg Clin North Am* 1991;2:807-816.

8. North RB, Kidd DH, Zahurak M, Piantadosi S: Specificity of diagnostic nerve blocks: A prospective, randomized study of sciatica due to lumbosacral spine disease. *Pain* 1996;65:77-85.

9. Deyo RA: Early diagnostic evaluation of low back pain. *J Gen Intern Med* 1986;1:328-338.

10. Deyo RA, Weinstein JN: Low back pain. *N Engl J Med* 2001,344:363-370.

11. Jarvik JG, Deyo RA: Diagnostic evaluation of low back pain with emphasis on imaging. *Ann Intern Med* 2002;137:586-597.

12. Deyo RA, Rainville J, Kent DL: What can the history and physical examination tell us about low back pain? *JAMA* 1992;268:760-765.

13. Wheeler AH: Diagnosis and management of low back pain and sciatica. *Am Fam Phys* 1995;52: 1333-1348.

14. Rigamonti D, Liem L, Sampath P, et al: Spinal epidural abscess: Contemporary trends in etiology, evaluation, and management. *Surg Neurol* 1999;52:189-197.

15. Broner FA, Garland DE, Zigler JE: Spinal infections in the immunocompromised host. *Orthop Clin North Am* 1996;27:37-46.

16. Prendergast H, Jerrard D, O'Connell J: Atypical presentations of epidural abscess in intravenous drug abusers. *Am J Emerg Med* 1997;15:158-160.

17. Koppel BS, Tuchman AJ, Mangiardi JR, Daras M, Weitzner I: Epidural spinal infection in intravenous drug abusers. *Arch Neurol* 1988;45:1331-1337.

18. Moffat NA: Spondylitis following urinary tract instrumentation. *J Urol* 1973;110:339.

19. Waddell G, McCulloch JA, Kummel E, Venner RM: Nonorganic physical signs in low-back pain. *Spine* 1980;5:117-125.

20. Main CJ, Waddell G: Behavioral responses to examination: A reappraisal of the interpretation of "nonorganic signs." *Spine* 1998;23:2367-2371.

21. Vaccaro AR, Ring D, Scuderi G, Cohen DS, Garfin SR: Predictors of outcome in patients with chronic back pain and low-grade spondylolisthesis. *Spine* 1997;22: 2030-2035.

22. Klekamp J, McCarty E, Spengler DM: Results of elective lumbar discectomy for patients involved in the workers' compensation system. *J Spinal Disord* 1998;11:277-282.

23. Franklin GM, Haug J, Heyer NJ, McKeefrey SP, Picciano JF: Outcome of lumbar fusion in Washington state workers' compensation. *Spine* 1994;19:1897-1904.

24. Katz JN, Dalgas M, Stucki G, et al: Degenerative lumbar spinal stenosis: Diagnostic value of the history and physical examination. *Arthritis Rheum* 1995;38:1236-1241.

25. Deyo RA, Loeser JD, Bigos SJ: Herniated lumbar intervertebral disk. *Ann Intern Med* 1990;112:598-603.

26. Brown MD, Gomez-Marin O, Brookfield KF, Li PS: Differential diagnosis of hip disease versus spine disease. *Clin Orthop* 2004;419:280-284.

27. Tortolani PJ, Carbone JJ, Quartararo LG: Greater trochanteric pain syndrome in patients referred to orthopedic spine specialists. *Spine J* 2002;2:251-254.

28. Calin A, Kaye B, Sternberg M, Antell B, Chan M: The prevalence and nature of back pain in an industrial complex: A questionnaire and radiographic and HLA analysis. *Spine* 1980;5:201-205.

29. Jarvik JJ, Hollingworth W, Heagerty P, Haynor DR, Deyo RA: The Longitudinal Assessment of Imaging and Disability of the Back (LAIDBack) Study: Baseline data. *Spine* 2001;26:1158-1166.

30. Sartoris DJ, Clopton P, Nemcek A, Dowd C, Resnick D: Vertebral-body collapse in focal and diffuse disease: Patterns of pathologic processes. *Radiology* 1986;160: 479-483.

31. Sartoris DJ, Andre M, Resnik CS, Resnick D, Resnick C: Trabecular bone density in the proximal femur: Quantitative CT assessment. Work in progress. *Radiology* 1986;160:707-712.

32. Deyo RA, Diehl AK: Cancer as a cause of back pain: Frequency, clinical presentation, and diagnostic strategies. *J Gen Intern Med* 1988;3:230-238.

33. Modic MT, Feiglin DH, Piraino DW, et al: Vertebral osteomyelitis: Assessment using MR. *Radiology* 1985;157:157-166.

34. Robbins SE, Morse MH: Is the acquisition of a separate view of the sacroiliac joints in the prone position justified in patients with back pain? *Clin Radiol* 1996;51:637-638.

35. Scavone JG, Latshaw RF, Weidner WA: Anteroposterior and lateral radiographs: An adequate lumbar spine examination. *AJR Am J Roentgenol* 1981;136:715-717.

36. Pitkanen MT, Manninen HI, Lindgren KA, Sihvonen TA, Airaksinen O, Soimakallio S: Segmental lumbar spine instability at flexion-extension radiography can be predicted by conventional radiography. *Clin Radiol* 2002;57:632-639.

37. Wood KB, Popp CA, Transfeldt EE, Geissele AE: Radiographic evaluation of instability in spondylolisthesis. *Spine* 1994;19:1697-1703.

38. Webster EW, Merrill OE: Radiation hazards: II. Measurements of gonadal dose in radiographic examinations. *N Engl J Med* 1957;257:811-819.

39. Antoku S, Russell WJ: Dose to the active bone marrow, gonads, and skin from roentgenography and fluoroscopy. *Radiology* 1971;101:669-678.

40. Espeland A, Baerheim A, Albrektsen G, Korsbrekke K, Larsen JL: Patients' views on importance and usefulness of plain radiography for low back pain. *Spine* 2001;26:1356-1363.

41. Deyo RA, Diehl AK: Lumbar spine films in primary care: Current use and effects of selective ordering criteria. *J Gen Intern Med* 1986;1:20-25.

42. Tallroth K: Plain CT of the degenerative lumbar spine. *Eur J Radiol* 1998;27:206-213.

43. Godersky JC, Erickson DL, Seljeskog EL: Extreme lateral disc herniation: Diagnosis by computed tomographic scanning. *Neurosurgery* 1984;14:549-552.

44. Firooznia H, Benjamin V, Kricheff II, Rafii M, Golimbu C: CT of lumbar spine disk herniation: Correlation with surgical findings. *AJR Am J Roentgenol* 1984;142:587-592.

45. Jackson RP, Cain JE Jr, Jacobs RR, Cooper BR, McManus GE: The neuroradiographic diagnosis of lumbar herniated nucleus pulposus: II. A comparison of computed tomography (CT), myelography, CT-myelography, and magnetic resonance imaging. *Spine* 1989;14:1362-1367.

46. Thornbury JR, Fryback DG, Turski PA, et al: Disk-caused nerve compression in patients with acute low-back pain: Diagnosis with MR, CT myelography, and plain CT. Radiology 1993;186:731-738. Erratum in: *Radiology* 1993;187:880.

47. Mikhael MA, Ciric I, Tarkington JA, Vick NA: Neuroradiological evaluation of lateral recess syndrome. *Radiology* 1981;140:97-107.

48. Hasegawa T, An HS, Haughton VM, Nowicki BH: Lumbar foraminal stenosis: Critical heights of the intervertebral discs and foramina. A cryomicrotome study in cadavera. *J Bone Joint Surg Am* 1995;77:32-38.

49. Grobler LJ, Robertson PA, Novotny JE, Pope MH: Etiology of spondylolisthesis: Assessment of the role played by lumbar facet joint morphology. *Spine* 1993;18:80-91.

50. Albeck MJ, Danneskiold-Samsoe B: Patient attitudes to myelography, computed tomography and magnetic resonance imaging when examined for suspected lumbar disc herniation. *Acta Neurochir (Wien)* 1995;133:3-6.

51. Hollis PH, Malis LI, Zappulla RA: Neurological deterioration after lumbar puncture below complete spinal subarachnoid block. *J Neurosurg* 1986;64:253-256.

52. Kikkawa I, Sugimoto H, Saita K, Ookami H, Nakama S, Hoshino Y: The role of Gd-enhanced three-dimensional MRI fast low-angle shot (FLASH) in the evaluation of symptomatic lumbosacral nerve roots. *J Orthop Sci* 2001;6:101-109.

53. Lane JI, Koeller KK, Atkinson JL: Enhanced lumbar nerve roots in the spine without prior surgery: Radiculitis or radicular veins? *AJNR Am J Neuroradiol* 1994;15:1317-1325.

54. Larde D, Mathieu D, Frija J, Gaston A, Vasile N: Spinal vacuum phenomenon: CT diagnosis and significance. *J Comput Assist Tomogr* 1982;6:671-676.

55. Resnick D, Niwayama G, Guerra J Jr, Vint V, Usselman J: Spinal vacuum phenomena: Anatomical study and review. *Radiology* 1981;139:341-348.

56. Modic MT, Steinberg PM, Ross JS, Masaryk TJ, Carter JR: Degenerative disk disease: Assessment of changes in vertebral body marrow with MR imaging. *Radiology* 1988;166:193-199.

57. Vital JM, Gille O, Pointillart V, et al: Course of Modic 1 six months after lumbar posterior osteosynthesis. *Spine* 2003;28:715-721.

58. Sandhu HS, Sanchez-Caso LP, Parvataneni HK, Cammisa FP Jr, Girardi FP, Ghelman B: Association between findings of provocative discography and vertebral end-plate signal changes as seen on MRI. *J Spinal Disord* 2000;13:438-443.

59. Braithwaite I, White J, Saifuddin A, Renton P, Taylor BA: Vertebral end-plate (Modic) changes on lumbar spine MRI: Correlation with pain reproduction at lumbar discography. *Eur Spine J* 1998;7:363-368.

60. Brant-Zawadzki M, Jensen M: Spinal nomenclature. *Spine* 1995;20:388-390.

61. Carragee EJ, Paragioudakis SJ, Khurana S: Lumbar high-intensity zone and discography in subjects without low back problems. *Spine* 2000;25:2987-2992.

62. Lam KS, Carlin D, Mulholland RC: Lumbar disc high-intensity zone: The value and significance of provocative discography in the determination of the discogenic pain source. *Eur Spine J* 2000;9:36-41.

63. Rankine JJ, Gill KP, Hutchinson CE, Ross ER, Williamson JB: The clinical significance of the high-intensity zone on lumbar spine magnetic resonance imaging. *Spine* 1999;24:1913-1920.

64. Boden SD, Davis DO, Dina TS, Patronas NJ, Wiesel SW: Abnormal magnetic-resonance scans of the lumbar spine in asymptomatic subjects: A prospective investigation. *J Bone Joint Surg Am* 1990;72:403-408.

65. Weishaupt D, Zanetti M, Hodler J, Boos N: MR imaging of the lumbar spine: Prevalence of intervertebral disk extrusion and sequestration, nerve root compression, end plate abnormalities, and osteoarthritis of the facet joints in asymptomatic volunteers. *Radiology* 1998;209:661-666.

66. Kent DL, Haynor DR, Larson EB, Deyo RA: Diagnosis of lumbar spinal stenosis in adults: A metaanalysis of

the accuracy of CT, MR, and myelography. *AJR Am J Roentgenol* 1992;158:1135-1144.

67. Modic MT, Masaryk TJ, Ross JS, Carter JR: Imaging of degenerative disk disease. *Radiology* 1988;168:177-186.

68. Ullrich CG, Binet EF, Sanecki MG, Kieffer SA: Quantitative assessment of the lumbar spinal canal by computed tomography. *Radiology* 1980;134:137-143.

69. Czervionke LF, Berquist TH: Imaging of the spine: Techniques of MR imaging. *Orthop Clin North Am* 1997;28:583-616.

70. Speciale AC, Pietrobon R, Urban CW, et al: Observer variability in assessing lumbar spinal stenosis severity on magnetic resonance imaging and its relation to cross-sectional spinal canal area. *Spine* 2002;27:1082-1086.

71. Weishaupt D, Schmid MR, Zanetti M, et al: Positional MR imaging of the lumbar spine: Does it demonstrate nerve root compromise not visible at conventional MR imaging? *Radiology* 2000;215:247-253.

72. Weishaupt D, Boxheimer L: Magnetic resonance imaging of the weight-bearing spine. *Semin Musculoskelet Radiol* 2003;7:277-286.

73. Gillams AR, Chaddha B, Carter AP: MR appearances of the temporal evolution and resolution of infectious spondylitis. *AJR Am J Roentgenol* 1996;166:903-907.

74. Smith AS, Weinstein MA, Mizushima A, et al: MR imaging characteristics of tuberculous spondylitis vs vertebral osteomyelitis. *AJR Am J Roentgenol* 1989;153:399-405.

75. Algra PR, Bloem JL, Tissing H, Falke TH, Arndt JW, Verboom LJ: Detection of vertebral metastases: Comparison between MR imaging and bone scintigraphy. *Radiographics* 1991;11:219-232.

76. Avrahami E, Tadmor R, Dally O, Hadar H: Early MR demonstration of spinal metastases in patients with normal radiographs and CT and radionuclide bone scans. *J Comput Assist Tomogr* 1989;13:598-602.

77. Carroll KW, Feller JF, Tirman PF: Useful internal standards for distinguishing infiltrative marrow pathology from hematopoietic marrow at MRI. *J Magn Reson Imaging* 1997;7:394-398.

78. An HS, Andreshak TG, Nguyen C, Williams A, Daniels D: Can we distinguish between benign versus malignant compression fractures of the spine by magnetic resonance imaging? *Spine* 1995;20:1776-1782.

79. Baur A, Stabler A, Bruning R, et al: Diffusion-weighted MR imaging of bone marrow: Differentiation of benign versus pathologic compression fractures. *Radiology* 1998;207:349-356.

80. Swanson D, Blecker I, Gahbauer H, Caride VJ: Diagnosis of discitis by SPECT technetium-99m MDP scintigram: A case report. *Clin Nucl Med* 1987;12:210-211.

81. Han LJ, Au-Yong TK, Tong WC, Chu KS, Szeto LT, Wong CP: Comparison of bone single-photon emission tomography and planar imaging in the detection of vertebral metastases in patients with back pain. *Eur J Nucl Med* 1998;25:635-638.

82. Maynard AS, Jensen ME, Schweickert PA, Marx WF, Short JG, Kallmes DF: Value of bone scan imaging in predicting pain relief from percutaneous vertebroplasty in osteoporotic vertebral fractures. *AJNR Am J Neuroradiol* 2000;21:1807-1812.

83. Beattie PF, Meyers SP, Stratford P, Millard RW, Hollenberg GM: Associations between patient report of symptoms and anatomic impairment visible on lumbar magnetic resonance imaging. *Spine* 2000;25:819-828.

84. Nardin RA, Patel MR, Gudas TF, Rutkove SB, Raynor EM: Electromyography and magnetic resonance imaging in the evaluation of radiculopathy. *Muscle Nerve* 1999;22:151-155.

85. Tsao BE, Levin KH, Bodner RA: Comparison of surgical and electrodiagnostic findings in single root lumbosacral radiculopathies. *Muscle Nerve* 2003;27:60-64.

86. Holt EP Jr: The question of lumbar discography. *J Bone Joint Surg Am* 1968;50:720-726.

87. Walsh TR, Weinstein JN, Spratt KF, Lehmann TR, Aprill C, Sayre H: Lumbar discography in normal subjects: A controlled, prospective study. *J Bone Joint Surg Am* 1990;72:1081-1088.

88. Carragee EJ, Tanner CM, Khurana S, et al: The rates of false-positive lumbar discography in select patients without low back symptoms. *Spine* 2000;25:1373-1381.

89. Carragee EJ, Tanner CM, Yang B, Brito JL, Truong T: False-positive findings on lumbar discography: Reliability of subjective concordance assessment during provocative disc injection. *Spine* 1999;24:2542-2547.

90. Derby R, Howard MW, Grant JM, Lettice JJ, Van Peteghem PK, Ryan DP: The ability of pressure-controlled discography to predict surgical and nonsurgical outcomes. *Spine* 1999;2:364-372.

91. Guyer RD, Ohnmeiss DD, NASS: Lumbar discography. *Spine J* 2003;3(suppl):11S-27S.

92. Smith SE, Darden BV, Rhyne AL, Wood KE: Outcome of unoperated discogram-positive low back pain. *Spine* 1995;20:1997-2001.

93. Colhoun E, McCall IW, Williams L, Cassar Pullicino VN: Provocation discography as a guide to planning operations on the spine. *J Bone Joint Surg Br* 1988;70:267-271.

94. Madan S, Gundanna M, Harley JM, Boeree NR, Sampson M: Does provocative discography screening of discogenic back pain improve surgical outcome? *J Spinal Disord Tech* 2002;15:245-251.

95. Mooney V, Robertson J: The facet syndrome. *Clin Orthop* 1976;115:149-156.

96. Helbig T, Lee CK: The lumbar facet syndrome. *Spine* 1988;13:61-64.

97. Revel M, Poiraudeau S, Auleley GR, et al: Capacity of the clinical picture to characterize low back pain relieved by facet joint anesthesia: Proposed criteria to identify patients with painful facet joints. *Spine* 1998;23:1972-1977.

98. Goldthwaith JE: The lumbosacral articulation: An explanation of many cases of lumbago, sciatica, and paraplegia. *Boston Med Surg J* 1911;164:365-372.

99. Schwarzer AC, Aprill CN, Derby R, Fortin J, Kine G, Bogduk N: Clinical features of patients with pain stemming from the lumbar zygapophysial joints: Is the lumbar facet syndrome a clinical entity? *Spine* 1994;19:1132-1137.

100. Schwarzer AC, Wang SC, O'Driscoll D, Harrington T, Bogduk N, Laurent R: The ability of computed tomography to identify a painful zygapophysial joint in patients with chronic low back pain. *Spine* 1995;20:907-912.

101. Bogduk N: International Spinal Injection Society guidelines for the performance of spinal injection procedures: Part 1. Zygapophysial joint blocks. *Clin J Pain* 1997;13:285-302.

102. Fukui S, Ohseto K, Shiotani M, Ohno K, Karasawa H, Naganuma Y: Distribution of referred pain from the lumbar zygapopheseal joints and dorsal rami. *Clin J Pain* 1997;13:303-307.

103. Moran R, O'Connell D, Walsh MG: The diagnostic value of facet joint injections. *Spine* 1988;13:1407-1410.

104. Dreyfuss P, Halbrook B, Pauza K, Joshi A, McLarty J, Bogduk N: Efficacy and validity of radiofrequency neurotomy for chronic lumbar zygapophysial joint pain. *Spine* 2000;25:1270-1277.

105. Esses SI, Moro JK: The value of facet joint blocks in patient selection for lumbar fusion.` *Spine* 1993;18:185-190.

106. Mersky H, Bogduk N: Spinal and radicular pain syndromes of lumbar, sacral, and coccygeal regions, in Mersky H, Bogduk N (eds): *Classification of Chronic Pain: Pain Descriptions of Chronic Pain Syndromes and Definition of Pain Terms*, ed 2. Seattle, WA, IASP Press, 1994, pp 190-191.

107. Fortin JD, Dwyer AP, West S, Pier J: Sacroiliac joint: pain referral maps upon applying a new injection/arthrography technique: Part I. Asymptomatic volunteers. *Spine* 1994;19:1475-1482.

108. Maigne JY, Aivaliklis A, Pfefer F: Results of sacroiliac joint double block and value of sacroiliac pain provocation tests in 54 patients with low back pain. *Spine* 1996;21:1889-1892.

109. Dreyfuss P, Dryer S, Griffin J, Hoffman J, Walsh N: Positive sacroiliac screening tests in asymptomatic adults. *Spine* 1994;19:1138-1143.

110. Schwarzer AC, Aprill CN, Bogduk N: The sacroiliac joint in chronic low back pain. *Spine* 1995;20:31-37.

111. Chou LH, Slipman CW, Bhagia SM, et al: Inciting events initiating injection-proven sacroiliac joint syndrome. *Pain Med* 2004;5:26-32.

112. Fortin JD: The sacroiliac joint: A new perspective. *Am J Back Musculoskel Rehab* 1993;3:31-43.

113. Dreyfuss P, Michaelsen M, Pauza K, McLarty J, Bogduk N: The value of medical history and physical examination in diagnosing sacroiliac joint pain. *Spine* 1996;21:2594-2602.

114. Slipman CW, Lipetz JS, Plastaras CT, et al: Fluoroscopically guided therapeutic sacroiliac joint injections for sacroiliac joint syndrome. *Am J Phys Med Rehabil* 2001;80:425-432.

115. Ferrante FM, King LF, Roche EA, et al: Radiofrequency sacroiliac joint denervation for sacroiliac syndrome. *Reg Anesth Pain Med* 2001;26:137-142.

CHAPTER 5

SURGICAL MANAGEMENT OF CHRONIC LOW BACK PAIN: ARTHRODESIS

SAMEER MATHUR, MD
LOUIS G. JENIS, MD
HOWARD S. AN, MD

Chronic low back pain (LBP), which is loosely defined as pain of more than 12 weeks' duration, evolves in a complex environment. Influenced by both internal and external factors, LBP results in pain and disability that alters a patient's function beyond what would be expected for the initiating pathologic dysfunction.[1,2] LBP is so prevalent that the Agency for Healthcare Research and Quality of the US Department of Health and Human Services developed and published national guidelines in 1994 to assist physicians in the appropriate care of affected patients.[3]

Despite its widespread prevalence, LBP is still an enigma, with a loosely defined diagnosis based on complex pathoanatomic issues. Evidence concerning its cause, proper management, and prognosis remains insufficient. The first scientific explanation for the source of low back and leg pain was presented in 1934, when Mixter and Barr[4] attributed back symptoms to prolapse of the intervertebral disk. Treatment remains complicated by the lack of correlation between pathologic physical findings and a patient's pain and disability.[1,5] In recent decades, numerous advancements in diagnostic and therapeutic modalities, including radiologic, electrodiagnostic, and injection techniques, have identified structural causes of LBP and directed treatment algorithms. This chapter reviews the options for surgical treatment of chronic LBP secondary to degenerative disk disease.

INDICATIONS

Spinal arthrodesis was first used for the treatment of infectious conditions, deformity, and trauma of the spine. However, technical advances in imaging, surgical procedures, implants, and bone grafting have expanded the indications for spinal arthrodesis in an attempt to control recalcitrant pain attributed to either abnormal or unstable motion between vertebrae or mechanical degeneration of the intervertebral disk.[5-7] Under ideal circumstances, spinal arthrodesis should be performed only after a specific pathoanatomic diagnosis is made in which the disk (discogenic back pain) or facet joints

FIGURE 1

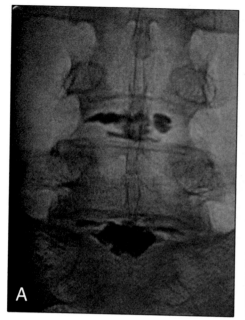

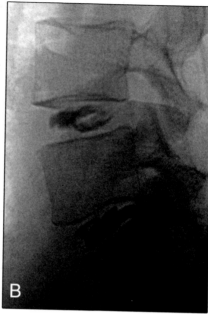

AP **(A)** and lateral **(B)** radiographs of the lumbar spine depicting contrast medium injected into the L4-5 and L5-S1 disk spaces during a diskogram. The dye increases the pressure in the disk to mimic the pressure of prolonged sitting or standing.

(facet syndrome) are identified as the most common sites of pain. The natural history of the condition also must be understood so that the timing of surgical intervention is appropriate.

Lumbar arthrodesis currently is a common treatment of LBP. In 2001, the Swedish Lumbar Spine Study Group conducted a prospective, randomized clinical trial comparing the efficacy of lumbar arthrodesis with nonsurgical treatment in reducing pain and decreasing disability in a group of 294 patients with chronic LBP resulting from degenerative disk disease but not spondylolisthesis.[8] At 2-year follow-up, patients who received surgical treatment were found to have better clinical and functional outcomes than patients who received nonsurgical treatment.

The indications for surgical treatment of patients with discogenic pain include disabling pain of more than 6 to 12 months' duration, failed nonsurgical therapy, and advanced disk degeneration evident on an MRI scan with a concordant positive diskogram (Figure 1). In addition, patients should not have psychosocial issues or secondary gains that could affect recovery. Currently, treatment of discogenic pain includes removing the disk, restoring disk height to reestablish the normal tension

in the anulus fibrosis, increasing lumbar lordosis, indirectly opening the neuroforamina, and stabilizing the motion segments[9-12] (Figure 2). In addition, fusion of the spinal motion segment eliminates the pain generated by facet joint arthropathy.

TECHNIQUES

Methods to achieve arthrodesis for the treatment of LBP include posterolateral arthrodesis alone, anterior disk excision and interbody fusion, posterior lumbar disk excision and interbody fusion, and circumferential stabilization procedures. Even though indications for a specific approach are lacking, most surgeons find that certain anatomic and patient characteristics will identify the most appropriate procedure for a given individual.

Posterolateral Arthrodesis

Posterolateral fusion with autogenous bone graft, with or without pedicle screw instrumentation, is commonly performed for numerous etiologies. If the fusion is successful, vertebral motion will be limited, thereby reduc-

FIGURE 2

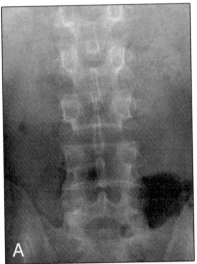 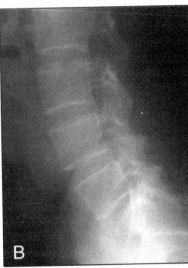 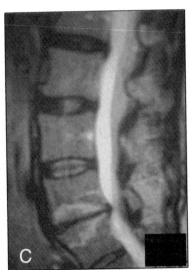

AP **(A)** and lateral **(B)** radiographs of the lumbar spine demonstrating mild changes at the L4-5 disk space and moderate to severe changes at the L5-S1 disk space. **C,** A T2-weighted MRI scan of the lumbar spine illustrating degenerative disk disease (dark disk) with end-plate changes.

ing the stimulus for pain. Hibbs,[13] in 1912, reported techniques for achieving posterolateral spinal fusion by placing bone graft directly on the lamina. Cleveland and associates,[14] in 1948, moved the bone graft more laterally to the intertransverse (posterolateral) plane based on the significant incidence of pseudarthrosis with central bone graft placement. The pseudarthrosis rate after posterolateral fusion ranges from approximately 5% to 45% and increases with the number of levels fused.[11,12,15,16]

Instrumentation, when used as an adjunct to posterolateral fusion, may confer immediate stability to the affected motion segment and decrease the rate of pseudarthrosis to 5%. In a prospective, randomized trial, Zdeblick[17] reported on 49 patients who underwent posterolateral fusion for chronic discogenic back pain. A total of 95% of their patients who underwent posterolateral fusion with pedicle instrumentation had good or excellent results compared with 71% of patients who had in situ fusion. Lorenz and associates[18] retrospectively reviewed the records of 47 patients who underwent single-level posterolateral fusion with and without instrumentation. Pseudarthrosis rates were 58% in patients who did not have instrumentation and 0% in patients who did (Figure 3). Many studies have docu-

mented the role of instrumentation in improving bone graft incorporation, although similar effects on clinical outcome vary.[19-22] Achieving radiographic fusion does not universally correlate with a successful clinical outcome, confirming the importance of appropriate diagnosis and patient selection.

Advantages of posterolateral fusion include the relative ease of the procedure and the ability to adequately decompress the neural elements while avoiding the potential pitfalls associated with an anterior approach. One significant disadvantage to the posterior approach and preparation of the posterolateral intertransverse area is the potential to damage the paraspinal musculature. The problem of "fusion disease" has been reported as a leading cause of continued postoperative pain from this approach.[23]

Clinical outcomes of this approach are mediocre at best, with good to excellent results ranging from approximately 40% to 80%, and likely relate to the pain generator[23] (Figure 4). Persistent discogenic back pain, despite a solid posterolateral fusion, has been documented, and preclinical studies have suggested that the biomechanically inferior position of the intertransverse graft may allow continued micromotion through the painful anterior column.[24] Persistent pain after posterior

FIGURE 3

FIGURE 4

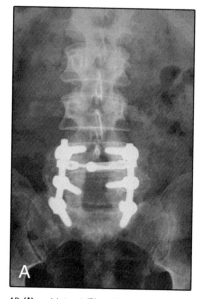 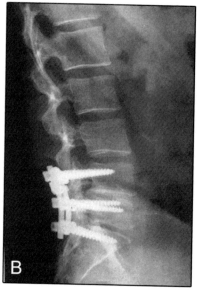

AP (A) and lateral (B) radiographs taken following posterolateral fusion with instrumentation.

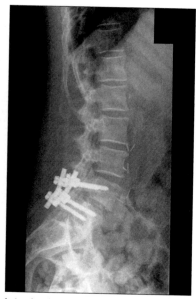

Lateral radiograph taken following PLIF with posterior pedicle screw fixation.

fusion for discogenic back pain may be treated with the addition of an interbody fusion.

Posterolateral fusion has a reasonable success rate in appropriately selected patients, and pedicle screw instrumentation appears to lower the rate of pseudarthrosis. The principal indication for posterolateral fusion may be LBP from a facet syndrome and/or a discogenic origin.

Lumbar Interbody Fusion

Reduced motion across the disk achieved with posterolateral fusion may not be sufficient to prevent diffusion of biochemical substances to the richly innervated peripheral anulus. A number of procedures eliminate the disk as a potential pain generator, specifically anterior lumbar interbody fusion (ALIF), posterior or transforaminal lumbar interbody fusion (PLIF or TLIF), and circumferential arthrodesis.[25,26]

Jaslow[27] originally reported excision of the intervertebral disk and lumbar interbody fusion in 1946 for the treatment of tuberculosis. Cloward[28] popularized the procedure for the treatment of axial LBP via a posterior approach. Excision of the disk and interbody fusion is thought to remove the source of pain and prevent motion. This procedure also restores intervertebral height and may require a smaller amount of bone graft than is needed for posterior fusion.[26-29]

Posterior Lumbar Interbody Fusion

PLIF is a technically demanding procedure that involves wide posterior bilateral decompression and complete excision of the disk. Retraction of the nerve root and thecal sac is required to expose the disk space. Through the posterior exposure, bone graft is placed anteriorly between contiguous vertebral bodies. Interbody disk containment devices (spacers) or cages may be used to distract the anterior column, restore disk height, and provide immediate stability. Numerous metal and synthetic cage alternatives have been developed, including threaded cylindrical, mesh, or carbon fiber rectangular devices. Posterior pedicle instrumentation is recommended to decrease the rate of pseudarthrosis and prevent graft dislodgement (Figure 5).

The advantages of PLIF include removal of the pain generator, restoration of disk height with an anterior bone graft, and complete nerve root decompression. Because the anterior column provides 80% of weight-

FIGURE 5

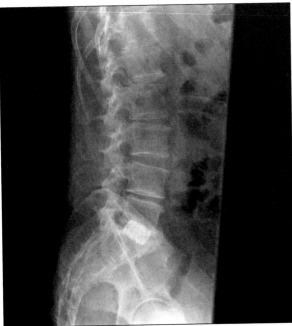

Lateral radiograph taken following ALIF with threaded cage instrumentation.

bearing support, there is increased biomechanical stability by placing an interbody device. Disadvantages include the need for significant retraction, possible injury to the nerve roots, dural tears, epidural scar formation, migration of interbody devices, fusion disease from muscle retraction, and pseudarthrosis.[17,26]

The radiographic results of PLIF confirm high fusion rates, and, when clinical outcomes specific to discogenic pain syndrome are evaluated, reasonable results are noted.[30,31] Schechter and associates[32] achieved good and excellent results in 89% of patients, with an overall fusion rate of 95%. Lin[26] reported good and excellent results in 86% of patients who underwent PLIF, with a 96% fusion rate. Fusion rates were similar across all these series; however, clinical outcomes were difficult to discern. Wetzel and LaRocca[33] reported failed PLIFs in which their patients reported persistent back and radicular pain from nerve tethering. The higher complication rate associated with postoperative recalcitrant nerve root pain appears to be the most important disadvantage to the use of PLIF in the absence of preoperative leg pain.[8]

Transforaminal Lumbar Interbody Fusion
TLIF is a variation of PLIF in which a unilateral facetectomy through a posterior approach is used to gain access to the disk space. Posterior distraction across the pedicle screws initially allows access to the disk and restores anterior column stability by insertion of a spacer that contains bone graft. Posterior compression restores the tension-band principle of the lumbar motion segment.[34]

The TLIF approach reduces risk of neurologic injury, provides a 360° fusion, avoids anterior spinal exposure and associated complications, reduces damage to ligamentous elements, minimizes excessive bone removal, and provides early mobilization. This approach also immobilizes the anterior column more effectively than posterolateral fusion, with or without instrumentation. Humphreys and associates,[35] investigating a retrospective series of patients who underwent PLIF or TLIF, reported a higher incidence of postoperative radiculitis in patients who had PLIF; however, clinical outcomes specific to degenerative disk disease were not reported.

The reported clinical outcomes of discogenic back pain managed by TLIF are limited. Hee and associates[36] reported reasonable improvements in pain in a retrospective series of patients who underwent TLIF.

Anterior Lumbar Interbody Fusion
ALIF involves an anterior approach to the lumbar spine, with complete excision of the disk and preparation of the end plates, which allows for exposure to cancellous surface for graft incorporation. The principal advantage of ALIF is direct removal of the involved disk, generally more complete than what can be achieved with PLIF. In addition, ALIF avoids damaging the posterior neural structures, iatrogenic trauma associated with posterior paraspinal muscle dissection, and partial denervation of the facet joints. ALIF also has disadvantages: the complexities associated with the anterior approach; the potential injury to the great vessels, intestines, bowel, or presacral plexus; and possible development of retrograde ejaculation.[37] An open, miniopen, or laparoscopic technique, which usually requires an approach surgeon for assistance, may be used for ALIF.

Either structural autograft or allograft can be inserted into the disk space. Implants that contain bone graft have several proposed advantages, including improved fusion rates, restoration and maintenance of disk height, and improved sagittal alignment.[38] Some implants may be used alone, whereas others require additional posterior fixation. The stand-alone implants (eg, threaded cages) depend on intersegmental distraction and tensioning of the lateral and posterior anulus, which provide immediate stability compared with traditional ALIF procedures (Figure 6).

Specific instruments have been developed for easier implant insertion. Lordotic or parallel spacers are used for distraction and reaming to create a channel for more accurate positioning of the implant. These devices contact the end plate and require that the cortical margins of the end plate be somewhat preserved to prevent subsidence. Threaded cages are titanium cylindrical devices with openings on the end plate side of the implant to allow for bone ingrowth; cages are available in parallel or lordotic configurations. Proponents of lordotic cages argue that this configuration allows for greater restoration of a lordotic disk space in the lower lumbar spine and more anatomic restoration of the sagittal contours.[38]

The use of supplemental posterior fixation depends on the presence of instability, spondylolisthesis, or lack of stability with the anterior construct. An implant without "teeth" or that is not threaded, such as an upright mesh cage, may not be considered as a stand-alone device.

Clinical outcomes and fusion rates following ALIF vary, depending on the number of levels to be fused, the types of implant used, and the use of allograft versus autogenous graft. Penta and Fraser[39] reported that 108 patients who underwent ALIF had a 68% fair or better outcome at 10-year follow-up. The fusion rate of a single-level arthrodesis was 91% but only 51% for multiple levels. In a different study of 150 patients who underwent ALIF, Greenough and associates[40] reported a fusion rate of 76% and a clinical success rate of 68%. Knox and Chapman,[41] who analyzed the results of 22 patients who had ALIF for degenerative disk disease, reported a lower success rate. Of the 17 patients who had a single-level arthrodesis, six had a good result, three had a fair result, and eight had a poor result. Outcomes of all five patients who had a two-level arthrodesis ranged from good to poor.[41] The best results appear to occur in the context of a thorough evaluation of the patient's condition, documentation of a specific pain generator in a discogenic syndrome and limiting surgery to one or two levels.[42-44]

FIGURE 6

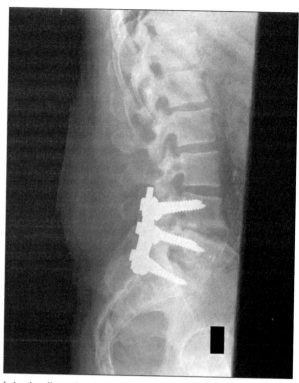

Lateral radiograph taken following ALIF and posterior fixation (360° fusion).

Circumferential Arthrodesis

Circumferential or 360° spinal arthrodesis was first used in the treatment of trauma and deformity. Following success in those scenarios, the indications were expanded to include axial back pain. The proponents of this technique claim that all potential sources of pain are eliminated, including anterior and posterior structures, and that stability is optimized. Pedicle screw instrumentation generally is used as an adjunct to posterior fusion in this procedure (Figure 6). The pseudarthrosis rate ranges from 5% to 10% for one- or two-level fusions.[15] Leufven and Nordwall[45] reported on 29 patients treated with instrumented PLIF and posterolateral fusion for disabling, chronic LBP. Solid fusion was obtained in 27 of 29 patients, and there was a significant reduction in back and leg pain. However, only 31% of the patients reported excellent results, whereas 27% had poor results, and 62% had not returned to work.

Minimally Invasive Techniques

Minimally invasive techniques have revolutionized the management of pathologic conditions in a number of surgical disciplines and recently have been applied to spine surgery. Conventional lumbar fusion techniques require extensive soft-tissue dissection for anatomic pedicle screw placement and for preparation of the fusion bed. Intraoperative tissue injury can increase postoperative pain, lengthen recovery time, and impair the spinal fusion by altering the local blood supply.

The results of minimally invasive ALIF techniques have been mixed. Laparoscopic transperitoneal ALIF was well received initially, but retrograde ejaculation caused by damage to the hypogastric plexus was a significant complication. In addition, bifurcation of the great vessels can impede exposure at the L4-5 level. The percentage of complications has ranged from 10% to 20%, but results of miniopen retroperitoneal ALIF appear to be better.[46-49]

A significant development in minimally invasive PLIF is a procedure in which 25-mm incisions are made over the disk space and the paraspinous muscles are dissected using a series of dilators under fluoroscopic guidance. A working tube of appropriate length is then placed at the lamina-facet junction over the disk space, and the procedure is performed directly through this conduit under direct visualization or magnification. A hemilaminotomy with medial facetectomy may be completed followed by an extensive diskectomy. The disk space is distracted, and various combinations of composite grafts (including cages) can be used. Subsequently, pedicle screws are placed through the same incision.[47,50]

TLIF also can be performed using a tube to perform a facetectomy to access the disk space. Distraction is achieved through the posterior elements, and supplemental pedicle screw fixation is added. TLIF can be performed through the tube dilator system (similarly to PLIF), but the skin incision is made 45 to 50 mm lateral to the midline. The contralateral incision can be used to insert percutaneous pedicle screws (Figure 7).

Preliminary results with minimally invasive spine surgery demonstrate that it can be done safely and effectively. However, there is a significant learning curve. Prospective long-term studies eventually will better define the role of minimally invasive surgery in the management of chronic LBP.

FIGURE 7

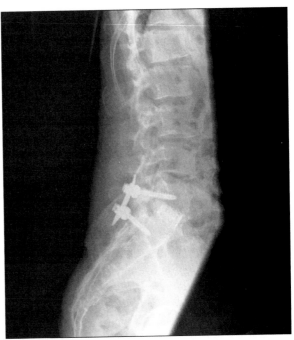

Lateral radiograph taken following TLIF and percutaneous posterior pedicle screw fixation.

CONCLUSION

On presentation, chronic LBP simply can be a constellation of signs and symptoms that often are not associated with any specific diagnosis. The physician must then evaluate the symptoms and results of physical examination and diagnostic testing to formulate an accurate diagnosis and prescribe appropriate therapy. Patients who have intractable pain, with one- or two-level disk degeneration confirmed by imaging, and concordant symptoms might be candidates for surgery. Few well-designed prospective, randomized clinical trials focus on the management of chronic LBP from degenerative disk disease; however, evidence exists that reasonable outcomes may be expected with specific patient selection and appropriate technique.

Numerous surgical approaches are available to treat degenerative LBP, each with advantages and disadvantages and varying degrees of technical difficulty. Fritzell and associates[46] reported results of a multicenter randomized study analyzing patients in three surgical groups: posterolateral fusion, posterolateral fusion combined with pedicle screw instrumentation, and postero-lateral fusion with interbody fusion (anterior and posterior). At 2-year follow-up, all groups reported reduced pain and disability, but the differences were not significant. In fact, there was no obvious disadvantage in using posterolateral fixation without internal fixation, considered the least demanding surgical technique. These results illustrate the point that surgical treatment of chronic LPB should be undertaken cautiously and only after appropriate discussion with the patient regarding alternatives and options for management. Additional research is required to further define the role of fusion in the management of chronic LBP.

REFERENCES

1. Brodke D, Ritter S: Nonoperative management of low back pain and lumbar disc degeneration. *J Bone Joint Surg Am* 2004;86:1810-1821.

2. Centeno C, Fleishman J: Degenerative disc disease and pre-existing spinal pain. *Ann Rheum Dis* 2003;62:371-372.

3. Bigos SJ, et al: *Acute Low Back Problems in Adults: Assessment and Treatment. Quick Reference Guide for Clinicians No. 14.* AHCPR Publication No 95-0643. Rockville, MD, Agency for Health Care Policy and Research, U.S. Department of Health and Human Services, 1994.

4. Mixter WJ, Barr JS: Rupture of the intervertebral disc with involvement of the spinal canal. *N Engl J Med* 1934;211:205-210.

5. Hanley E, David S: Lumbar arthrodesis for the treatment of back pain. *J Bone Joint Surg Am* 1999;81:716-730.

6. Katz J: Lumbar spine fusion: Surgical rates, costs, and complications. *Spine* 1995;20(suppl):78-83.

7. Kuslich SD, Danielson G, Dowdle JD, et al: Four-year follow-up results of lumbar spine arthrodesis using the Bagby and Kuslich lumbar fusion cage. *Spine* 2000;25:2656-2662.

8. Fritzell P, Hagg O, Wessberg P, Nordwall A: Lumbar fusion versus nonsurgical treatment for chronic low back pain: A multicenter randomized controlled trial from the Swedish Lumbar Spine Study Group. *Spine* 2001;26:2521-2532.

9. Lanman T, Hopkins T: Lumbar interbody fusion after treatment with recombinant human bone morpho-genetic protein-2 added to poly(L-lactide-co-D,L-lactide) bioresorbable implants. *Neurosurg Focus* 2004;16:E9.

10. Madan S, Harley J, Boeree N: Circumferential and posterolateral fusion for lumbar disc disease. *Clin Orthop* 2003;409:114-123.

11. Mirovsky Y, Halperin N, Anekstein Y, Neuwirth MG: Good results of circumferential spine fusion in smokers, using autograft and allograft. *Cell Tissue Bank* 2002;3:169-173.

12. Sengupta DK: Dynamic stabilization devices in the treatment of low back pain. *Orthop Clin North Am* 2004;35:43-56.

13. Hibbs RA: An operation for Pott's disease of the spine. *JAMA* 1912;9:842-851.

14. Cleveland M, Bosworth DM, Thompson FR: Pseud-arthrosis in lumbosacral spine. *J Bone Joint Surg Am* 1948;30:302-312.

15. Bono C, Lee C: Critical analysis of trends in fusion for degenerative disc disease over the past 20 years: Influence of technique on fusion rate and clinical outcome. *Spine* 2004;29:455-463.

16. Waddell G: Low back pain: A twentieth century health care enigma. *Spine* 1996;21:2820-2825.

17. Zdeblick T: A prospective, randomized study of lumbar fusion: Preliminary results. *Spine* 1993;18:983-991.

18. Lorenz M, Zindrick M, Schwaegler P, et al: A comparison of single-level fusions with and without hardware. *Spine* 1991;16(8 suppl):S455-S458.

19. Yuan H, Garfin S, Dickman C, Mardjetko S: A historical cohort of pedicle screw fixation in thoracic, lumbar and sacral spinal fusion. *Spine* 1994;19(20 suppl): 2279S-2296S.

20. Wood G, Boyd R, Carothers T, et al: The effect of pedicle screw/plate fixation on lumbar/lumbosacral autogenous bone graft fusions in patients with degenerative disc disease. *Spine* 1995;29:819-880.

21. Thomsen K, Christensen F, Eiskjaer S, et al: The effect of pedicle screw instrumentation on functional outcome and fusion rates in posterolateral lumbar spinal fusion: A prospective, randomized, clinical study. *Spine* 1997;22:2813-2822.

22. France JC, Yaszemski MJ, Lauermann WC, et al: A randomized prospective study of posterolateral lumbar fusion: Outcomes with and without pedicle screw instrumentation. *Spine* 1999;24:553-560.

23. Kwon B, Vaccaro A, Grauer J: Indications, techniques, and outcomes of posterior surgery for chronic low back pain. *Orthop Clin North Am* 2003;34:297-308.

24. Weatherly C, Prickett C, O'Brien J: Discogenic pain persisting despite solid posterior fusion. *J Bone Joint Surg Br* 1986;68:142-143.

25. Haid RW Jr, Branch CL Jr, Alexander JT, Barkus JK: Posterior lumbar interbody fusion using recombinant

human bone morphogenetic protein type 2 with cylindrical interbody cages. *Spine J* 2004;4:527-538.

26. Lin PM: Posterior lumbar interbody fusion (PLIF): Past, present, and future. *Clin Neurosurg* 2000;47:470-482.

27. Jaslow IA: Intercorporeal bone graft in spinal fusion after disc removal. *Surg Gynecol Obstet* 1946;82:215-218.

28. Cloward RB: The treatment of ruptured lumbar intervertebral discs by vertebral body fusion: I. Indications, operative techniques, after care. *J Neurosurg* 1953;10:154-168.

29. Gunzburg R, Szpalski M, Andersson G: *Degenerative Disc Disease.* Philadelphia, PA, Lippincott Williams & Wilkins, 2004.

30. Lee C, Vessa P, Lee J: Chronic disabling low back pain syndrome caused by internal disc derangements: The results of disc excision and posterior lumbar interbody fusion. *Spine* 1995;20:356-361.

31. Brantigan J, Steffee A, Lewis M, Quinn L, Persenaire J: Lumbar interbody fusion using the Brantigan I/F cage for posterior lumbar interbody fusion and the variable pedicle screw placement system: Two year results from a Food and Drug Administration investigational device exemption clinical trial. *Spine* 2000;25:1437-1446.

32. Schechter N, France M, Lee C: Painful internal disc derangements of the lumbosacral spine: Discographic diagnosis and treatment by posterior lumbar interbody fusion. *Orthopedics* 1991;14:447-451.

33. Wetzel FT, LaRocca H: The failed posterior lumbar interbody fusion. *Spine* 1991;16:839-845.

34. Rosenberg W, Mummanemi P: Transforaminal lumbar interbody fusion: Technique, complications, and early results. *Neurosurg* 2001;48:569-574.

35. Humphreys C, Hodges S, Patwardhan A, Eck J, Murphy R, Covington L: Comparison of posterior and transforaminal approaches to lumbar interbody fusion. *Spine* 2001;26:567-571.

36. Hee H, CastroF, Majd M, Holt R, Myers L: Anterior/posterior lumbar fusion versus transforaminal lumbar interbody fusion: Analysis of complications and predictive factors. *J Spinal Disord* 2001;14:533-540.

37. Sasso R, Burkus J, LeHuec J: Retrograde ejaculation after anterior lumbar interbody fusion: Transperitoneal versus retroperitoneal exposure. *Spine* 2003;28:1023-1026.

38. Burkus J, Schuler T, Gornet M, Zdeblick T: Anterior lumbar interbody fusion for the management of

39. Penta M, Fraser R: Anterior lumbar interbody fusion. A minimum 10-year follow-up. *Spine* 1997;22:2429-2434.

40. Greenough C, Taylor L, Fraser R: Anterior lumbar fusion: Results, assessment techniques and prognostic factors. *Eur Spine J* 1994;3:225-230.

41. Knox B, Chapman T: Anterior lumbar interbody fusion for discogram concordant pain. *J Spinal Disord* 1993;6:242-244.

42. Kuslich S, Ulstrom C, Griffith S, Ahern J, Dowdle J: The Bagby and Kuslich method of lumbar interbody fusion: History, technique and 2-year follow-up results of a United States prospective, multicenter trial. *Spine* 1998;23:1267-1279.

43. Leong J, Chun S, Grange J, Fang D: Long-term results of lumbar intervertebral disc prolapse. *Spine* 1983;8:793-799.

44. Blumenthal S, Baker J, Doseett A, Selby D: The role of anterior lumbar fusion for internal disc disruption. *Spine* 1988;13:566-569.

45. Leufven C, Nordwall A: Management of chronic disabling low back pain with 360 degrees fusion: Results from pain provocation test and concurrent posterior lumbar interbody fusion, posterolateral fusion, and pedicle screw instrumentation in patients with chronic disabling low back pain. *Spine* 1999;24:2042-2045.

46. Fritzell P, Hagg O, Wessberg P: Chronic low back and fusion: A comparison of three surgical techniques. A prospective multicenter randomized study from the Swedish Lumbar Spine Study Group. *Spine* 2002;27:1131-1141.

47. An H, Andersson G, Lieberman I, Riew D, Transfeldt E: Minimally invasive surgery for lumbar degenerative disorders: Part II. Degenerative disc disease and lumbar stenosis. *Am J Orthop* 2000;29:937-942.

48. Chung SK, Lee SH, Lim SR, et al: Comparative study of laparoscopic L5-S1 fusion versus open mini-ALIF, with a minimum 2-year follow-up. *Eur Spine J* 2003;12:613-617.

49. Escobar E, Transfeldt E, Garvey C, Ogilvie J, Gruber J, Schultz L: Video-assisted versus open anterior lumbar spine fusion surgery: A comparison of four techniques and complications in 135 patients. *Spine* 2003;28:729-732.

50. Foley K, Holly L, Schwender J: Minimally invasive lumbar fusion. *Spine* 2003;28:S26-S35.

chronic low back pain: Current strategies and concepts. *Orthop Clin North Am* 2004;35:25-32.

CHAPTER 6

SURGICAL MANAGEMENT OF CHRONIC LOW BACK PAIN: ALTERNATIVES TO ARTHRODESIS

LOUIS G. JENIS, MD

The conventional treatment of chronic low back pain (LBP) has been nonsurgical, with standard regimens of medications, exercise and physical therapy, activity modification, and injection therapy. Surgical arthrodesis remains the gold standard for treating patients who fail to respond to prolonged nonsurgical treatment. Spinal fusion has been performed for decades, and a variety of approaches and techniques have evolved, with recent developments focusing on limiting associated tissue injury by insertion of minimally invasive devices and use of potent osteoinductive factors to achieve successful arthrodesis. Despite these significant advances in technology, the clinical improvement in pain does not appear to follow a similar path.

Bono and Lee[1] reviewed the literature from the last 20 years and found 78 reports on 4,454 patients who had had fusion for associated back pain symptoms. They reported an overall success rate of 75% but did not identify a significant trend toward improved outcomes with contemporary surgical approaches to LBP.

The clinical and radiographic outcomes of surgical fusion for chronic LBP vary depending on a number of factors, specifically the following: (1) the number of levels addressed; (2) the diagnosis; (3) whether the anatomic approach is anterior, posterior, or combined; (4) the use of instrumentation; and (5) the patient's socioeconomic status, including active workers' compensation, personal injury, or disability claims. In addition, successful arthrodesis in a degenerative lumbar motion segment does not correlate universally with an improved clinical outcome. The Swedish Lumbar Spine Study Group conducted a multicenter randomized study of 211 patients treated with lumbar fusion by three different surgical techniques and reported that the incidence of complications ranged from 12% to 40%.[2] Although no association between clinical outcome and complications was reported, the risk of a complication rose with increasing technical demand in a given procedure.

Because of the risk of early and late complications and the variability of clinical outcomes associated with fusion for chronic LBP, other treatment options have been investigated. This chapter reviews the literature and

FIGURE 1

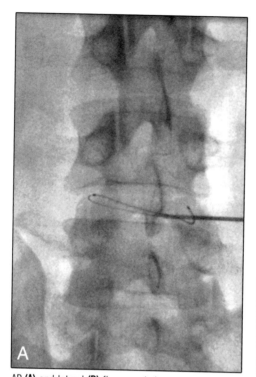 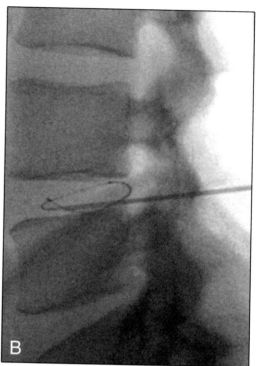

AP **(A)** and lateral **(B)** fluoroscopic images showing placement of the catheter coiled into the posterior anulus.

describes techniques and evidence that may be considered when managing a patient with chronic LBP.

INTERVERTEBRAL THERMAL THERAPIES

The concept of thermal therapy of the degenerated lumbar intervertebral disk is based on the use of radiofrequency (RF) to alter or shorten collagen fibers in capsulorrhaphy procedures in the peripheral joints. This minimally invasive technique may be directed at pathology originating from the anulus fibrosus or nucleus pulposus. Saal and Saal[3] developed a thermal resistive coil for insertion into a lumbar disk where it releases heat to repair annular defects. A flexible-tip catheter is coiled into the disk percutaneously under fluoroscopy while the patient is under conscious sedation (Figure 1). The heat is applied in slowly increasing increments to an area near the posterior anulus, which is a highly innervated region within the disk, and the annular tear or injury to

undergo repair, denervation, and eventual collagen fiber shortening and stabilization.[4] This technique of annuloplasty is also referred to as intradiskal electrothermal therapy or IDET (Oratec, Menlo Park, CA), and several clinical studies have been reported. Saal and Saal[5,6] reported on a prospective series of 62 patients with unremitting discogenic LBP treated by IDET. At 16-month (mean) follow-up, 71% of patients reported improvement in pain and functional outcome that appeared to be maintained at later evaluation. Other independent investigators, however, have been unable to confirm these results.[4] IDET appears relatively safe, with few procedural complications reported. Long-term data still are lacking, but analysis has suggested that the best clinical results are likely to occur in patients with a nearly intact anulus, significant preservation of disk height, and annular lesions localized to a small area in the posterior region.[7] Other forms of thermal annuloplasty have been developed and are under investigation (discTRODE, Radionics, Burlington, MA).

Thermal annuloplasty techniques remain controversial based on the variability of temperature changes within the anulus. Kleinstueck and associates,[8] reporting on cadaveric studies using IDET, found insufficient temperature changes to alter collagen architecture and a slight increase (10%) in motion indicative of mild instability after treatment. Histologic analysis is lacking; however, improvement in pain following these techniques is believed to be related to nociceptor denervation, although whether denervation is the sole mechanism of action remains in question.

PERCUTANEOUS NUCLEOTOMY AND NUCLEOPLASTY

Early disk degeneration is manifested as loss of hydration of the nucleus with disk height collapse. As the disk collapses and intradiskal pressure increases, annular bulging increases and may stretch nociceptive fibers within the outer layers of the anulus. The theory that LBP results from a disk bulge has led to the investigation of techniques that would reverse or limit the hoop stresses placed on the anulus by a degenerating nucleus. Decompression of the nucleus by nucleotomy or nucleoplasty has been described as a means of releasing the pressure on the highly innervated posterior anulus.[4]

Nucleoplasty relies on a localized field energy created by bipolar RF placed within the altered structures (Arthrocare Perc-D Coblation Spine Wand, Sunnyvale, CA). The procedure typically is performed while the patient is under local anesthesia with sedation, and fluoroscopic guidance is used for placing the probe in the appropriate position. Tissue within the disk is dissolved with minimal heat production and surrounding damage. Several passes of the probe into the nucleus create channels for decompression and further reduce disk volume. Series of patients in cohort-type studies have been reported to have acceptable clinical results at early follow-up.[9,10] However, randomized, prospective studies will be necessary for this technique to become a standard treatment for back pain.

Other forms of percutaneous removal of the nucleus have been used for several years. Automated percutaneous lumbar diskectomy, which is indicated only for contained, smaller-sized disk herniation or bulge, has been used for disk removal since 1984.[11] A probe is placed through a cannula and used to aspirate and debulk disk tissue. Clinical efficacy, however, remains variable, with success rates ranging from 29% to 80%, and the technique is performed by few investigators.[12-14] Disk tissue also may be debulked using laser energy to vaporize the nucleus and decrease intradiskal pressure; however, thermal injury to surrounding structures, including the adjacent anulus, nerve root, or cartilaginous end plate, is a risk. Clinical results are variable, and the use of laser therapy to manage LBP is limited.[15,16]

DYNAMIC STABILIZATION DEVICES

The lack of consistently successful clinical results with spinal fusion for LBP has led to the development of procedures for stabilizing the degenerative segment without associated arthrodesis. Dynamic or soft-tissue stabilization significantly lowers load transmission to the lumbar motion segment but does not eliminate motion and may restore a more physiologic loading pattern or prevent any abnormal motion.[17] The basic types of dynamic stabilization devices currently under clinical investigation include those placed between the spinous processes as distraction implants (Wallis system [Abbott Spine, Austin, TX]; X STOP [St. Francis Medical Technologies, Concord, CA]) or synthetic flexible ligaments attached to pedicle screw devices (Graf ligament [Surgicraft Limited, Worcestershire, UK]; Dynesis device [Zimmer Spine, Minneapolis, MN]). Several other forms of soft-tissue stabilization currently are in development but not yet available. Proponents of dynamic stabilization have claimed a few theoretical advantages, including maintaining flexibility to reduce loads on adjacent levels and providing the opportunity for disk repair by unloading the disk at the level of interest. Randomized clinical studies comparing outcomes of these devices to those for spinal fusion have not been published.

The interspinous devices distract and are loosely anchored to the spinous processes. The Wallis implant consists of a polyetheretherketone spacer and is currently being investigated in randomized clinical trials for the management of LBP.[18] The X STOP device is a titanium implant inserted between the spinous processes with the patient under a local anesthetic and is currently undergoing a US Food and Drug Administration (FDA) trial for treatment of symptoms related to spinal stenosis.

FIGURE 2

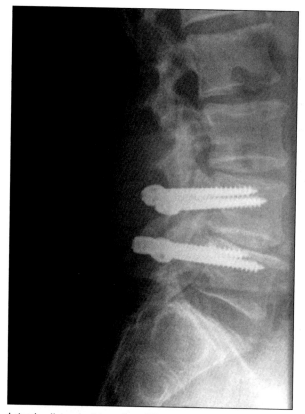

Lateral radiograph of dynamic stabilization implants (Dynesis device).

Several devices use ligaments attached across the pedicle screws for stabilization. The Graf ligament consists of nonelastic braided polyester looped around the pedicle screws and serves to lock the lumbar segment in extension to prevent rotatory instability.[19] This device is commonly used in the management of LBP outside of the United States, with outcomes similar to those for spinal fusion.[20-23] A potential complication of this device is possible exacerbation or creation of lateral recess stenosis during extension. Prophylactic decompression should be considered in patients in whom significant facet hypertrophy has been noted on preoperative imaging studies.

A dynamic neutralization system or Dynesis device is a similar type of construct with polyester cords and modular polycarbonaturethane spacers attached to the pedicle screws[24] (Figure 2). The spacers resist compressive forces between the screw heads while the cords decrease tensile loads. Positioning of the device, including the size of the spacers, is critical to establish segmental lordosis and load sharing within the construct and has been shown to correlate with clinical parameters.[18]

ARTIFICIAL DISK REPLACEMENT

Disk replacement technology has developed over the last 40 years. Most devices exist as theoretical alternatives to fusion, and very few have undergone in vivo testing or reached clinical study. A significant obstacle to the development of an artificial lumbar disk replacement has been the complexity of replicating the design and function of a normal anulus and nucleus. The replacement must allow for normal biomechanical and kinematic function of the anterior and posterior columns of the spine and withstand high compressive and shear loads for a lifespan that is equivalent to 50 to 100 million load cycles. For motion to be restored, the pain generator must be limited to the disk space, and evaluation of the facet joints must become a critical aspect of the diagnostic workup of LBP. The key design features of current disk technology include artificial nucleus and total disk replacement (TDR) and constraint of the implanted device.

Artificial Nucleus Replacement

The initial attempts to design artificial nucleus replacement devices focused on biomechanical replication of spine function. The goal was to restore annular tension and disk height through an open technique by removing and replacing the nucleus. Initial clinical studies in the 1950s used polymethylmethacrylate or self-curing silicone injected into the space occupied by the nucleus. These implants were limited by the ability to control the flow and curing rate of these substances and were abandoned. In 1966, Fernstrom[25] inserted spherical stainless-steel ball bearings in 125 patients at 191 lumbar or cervical levels. Although this procedure led to initial clinical improvement, eventual high stress loads on the cartilaginous end plates led to subsidence and disk collapse with recurrence of pain and to migration of the endoprosthesis through the annular defect used to insert the device.

With the development of biomaterials more appropriate for disk function, nuclear replacement technology has evolved to development of a device that reestablishes both biomechanical and biologic functions. Hydrogels consist of different compositions of polyvinyl alcohols (PVA), and the water-absorbing capacity of these structures can be adjusted by varying the ratio of hydrophilic and nonhydrophilic copolymers. The hydrophilic and viscoelastic properties of these hydrogels are remotely similar to those of normal disk tissue, and the hydrogels have been found to be capable of simulating in vitro biomechanical functions.

In 1988, Ray and Corbin developed a nuclear replacement device (Prosthetic Disc Nucleus, [PDN] Raymedica, Bloomington, MN) that consists of a PVA enclosed in an outer polyethylene jacket[26] (Figure 3). These semipermeable woven jackets are implanted in a dehydrated state through a posterior or anterolateral approach. The hydrogel's affinity for water causes the device to swell and theoretically locks the implant in place where it has been positioned. The structure becomes an incompressible bearing that expands on load application and transmits forces to surrounding structures. Nonrandomized studies of the PDN replacement device have reported improvement of clinical symptoms at 2-year follow-up in addition to restoration of sustained disk height.[27,28] Several iterations of the device have been developed over the last several years. Complications associated with the use of the PDN continue to relate to implant extrusion, which occurs in 12% to 26% of patients.[27]

Theoretical advantages of hydrogels include the ability to occupy a space determined by preexisting shape (ie, the hydrogel conforms to the space in a lock and key fashion), greater distribution of stress to the anulus and end plates, and less mechanical injury or annulotomy required during insertion. Numerous hydrogel devices are currently being developed for clinical considerations (Prosthetic Intervertebral Nucleus, Disc Dynamics, Eden Prairie, MN; BioDisc, CryoLife, Kennesaw, GA).

The critical issues surrounding the development of future nuclear replacement devices include delineation of their indications and insertion techniques.[26] If the device is oversized, extrusion is likely, and initial placement would be more difficult. An undersized implant would lead to less than optimal restoration of biomechanical properties, and, if unmatched within the disk space, uneven stress loads would be unlikely to lead to clinical improvement.

FIGURE 3

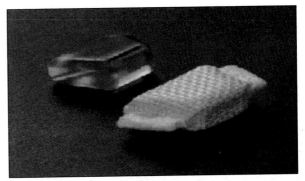

Nuclear replacement device (Prosthetic Disc Nucleus).

Total Disk Replacement

TDR devices allow for substitution of the anulus and nucleus components of the disk. Hinged or spring-loaded devices, devices with low-friction sliding surface, and devices with constrained fluid-filled chambers have been described.[29-31] Several contemporary designs have been developed that differ by the use of metal or plastic articulating surfaces, constraint of the implant, and attachment features. In 2004, the FDA released the Charite artificial disk replacement device (DePuy Spine, Raynham, MA) following an investigational device exempt (IDE) study. The study compared the safety and clinical and radiographic effectiveness of the Charite disk versus an anterior lumbar interbody fusion using BAK (Zimmer Spine) threaded cages packed with autogenous iliac crest graft[32-34] (P MacAfee and associates, unpublished data presented at the International Society for the Study of the Lumbar Spine annual meeting, 2004). The results showed that the clinical outcomes of improvement in pain and disability occurred early, continued through 24-month follow-up, and were similar in both groups. Greater patient satisfaction in the TDR group may have been related to the lack of requirement for postoperative bracing or restrictions normally applied to patients after fusion. There were few instances of minor displacement of the Charite disk but no reported instances of significant dislocation of the device. Radiographic evaluation revealed that both range of motion and disk height were maintained at follow-up, and implant positioning correlated with outcome (P MacAfee and associates, unpublished data pre-

FIGURE 4

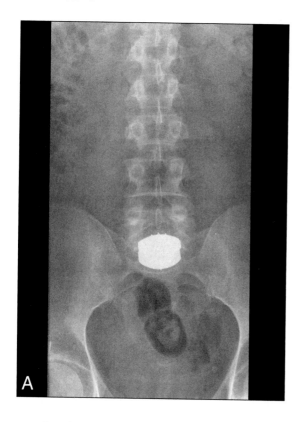

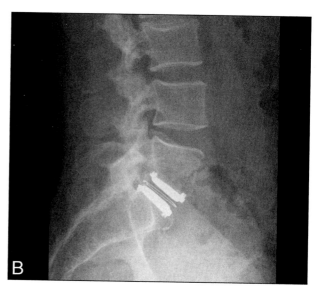

AP **(A)** and lateral **(B)** radiographs of Charite artificial disk replacement.

sented at the International Society for the Study of the Lumbar Spine annual meeting, 2004).

The Charite disk has gone through several iterations and currently consists of two cobalt-chrome end plates of various sizes and degrees of lordosis with six spikes on the undersurface of each end plate for early fixation (Figure 4). The concave superior and inferior articulating surfaces of the end plates contact a sliding nonconstrained ultra-high molecular weight polyethylene (UHMWPE) mobile core. In vitro and in vivo investigative studies have revealed the theoretical advantage of this type of articulating surface, which more closely matches the kinematics of the normal lumbar motion segment.[35] The mobile core simulates the translation of the nucleus during rotation and directs facet motion through a more normal pattern. The device is implanted through an anterior approach and requires precise positioning for restoration of normal kinematics.

Several other TDR devices currently are under investigation. These devices differ from the Charite TDR by the absence of a sliding mobile core and function more as a ball-and-socket type articulation. The ProDisc (Synthes, Paoli, PA) is a three-component device with a nonmobile UHMWPE spherical articulation snap-fit onto cobalt-chrome end plates. Lordosis is achieved through the superior end plate, and a midline keel fixes the end plates to the vertebral bodies. Marnay first implanted the ProDisc in 1990, and it is currently being investigated in one- or two-level degenerative disk disease in an FDA IDE study randomized to anterior-posterior lumbar fusion[36-38] (T Marnay, unpublished material presented at the North American Spine Society annual meeting, 2002). The Maverick Disc (Medtronics, Memphis, TN) and Flexicore Disc (Stryker, Allendale, NJ) replacement designs are metal-on-metal two-component designs currently under investigation. The former is attached by a midline keel, whereas the latter has a plasma-coated titanium spray with a bioactive hydroxyapatite layer for ingrowth.

Spinal arthroplasty is currently in its infancy and will develop over the next several decades. The critical issues that will need extensive investigation to determine the utility and indications for disk replacement technology are likely to include further identification of the pain generator so that patients may be included or excluded based on individual pathologies, ie, facet arthropathy. The positioning of these devices must be accurate because placement appears to affect outcome, and techniques that will enhance insertion are likely to be developed. Finally, spinal arthroplasty, just as peripheral joint arthroplasty, will likely have a defined lifespan based on wear of the articulating surfaces or development of the normal progression of facet disease that will require revision surgery. Whether revision surgery will involve removal of the anterior interbody device or placement of a posterior implant remains unresolved but is likely to be an important topic for discussion.

CONCLUSIONS

The goal of arthrodesis for chronic LBP is to eliminate motion at the lumbar segment in question with the potential short- and long-term drawbacks associated with these techniques. The search for alternatives to fusion has revealed options ranging from thermal ablation techniques that modify the annular collagen fibers to implants that minimize motion without associated fusion to disk replacement. These techniques are likely to be defined further in the future but will require extensive investigation, including prospective, randomized clinical trials to determine their effectiveness.

REFERENCES

1. Bono CM, Lee CK: Critical analysis of trends in fusion for degenerative disc disease over the past 20 years: Influence of technique on fusion rate and clinical outcome. *Spine* 2004;29:455-465.

2. Fritzell P, Hagg O, Nordwall A: Complications in lumbar fusion surgery for chronic low back pain: A comparison of three surgical techniques used in a prospective randomized study. A report from the Swedish Lumbar Spine Study Group. *Eur Spine J* 2003;12:178-189.

3. Saal JS, Saal JA: Management of chronic discogenic low back pain with a thermal intradiscal catheter: A preliminary report. *Spine* 2000;25:382-388.

4. Davis T, Sra P, Fuller N, Bae H: Lumbar intervertebral thermal therapies. *Orthop Clin North Am* 2003;34:255-262.

5. Saal JA, Saal JS: Intradiscal electrothermal treatment for chronic discogenic low back pain: A prospective outcome study with minimum 1-year follow-up. *Spine* 2000;25:2622-2627.

6. Saal JA, Saal JS: Intradiscal electrothermal treatment for chronic discogenic low back pain: A prospective outcome study with minimum 2-year follow-up. *Spine* 2002;27:966-973.

7. Karasek M, Bogduk N: Twelve-month follow-up of a controlled trial of intradiscal thermal annuloplasty for back pain due to internal disc disruption. *Spine* 2000;25:2601-2607.

8. Kleinstueck F, Diedrerich C, Nau W, et al: Acute biomechanical and histological effects of intradiscal electrothermal therapy on human lumbar discs. *Spine* 2001;26:2198-2207.

9. Sharps I, Issac Z: Percutaneous disc decompression using nucleoplasty. *Pain Phys* 2002;5:121-126.

10. Singh V, Piryani C, Liao K, et al: Percutaneous disc decompression using coblation (nucleoplasty) in the treatment of chronic discogenic pain. *Pain Phys* 2002;5:250-259.

11. Onik G, Helms C, Ginsburg L, Hoaglund F, Morris J: Percutaneous lumbar discectomy using a new aspiration probe. *AJR Am J Roentgenol* 1985;144:1137-1140.

12. Chatterjee S, Foy P, Findaly G: Report of a controlled clinical trial comparing automated percutaneous lumbar discectomy and microdiscectomy in the treatment of contained lumbar disc herniation. *Spine* 1995;20:734-738.

13. Revl M, Payan C, Vallee C, et al: Automated percutaneous lumbar discectomy versus chemonucleolysis in the treatment of sciatica: A randomized multicenter trial. *Spine* 1993;18:1-7.

14. Bonaldi G: Automated percutaneous lumbar discectomy: Technique, indications and clinical follow-up in over 1000 patients. *Neuroradiology* 2003;45:735-743.

15. Chen Y, Derby R, Lee S: Percutaneous disc decompression in the management of chronic low back pain. *Orthop Clin North Am* 2004;35:17-23.

16. Bosacco S, Bosacco D, Berman A, Cordover A, Levenberg R, Stell R: Functional results of percutaneous laser discectomy. *Am J Orthop* 1996;25:825-828.

17. Sengupta D: Dynamic stabilization devices in the treatment of low back pain. *Orthop Clin North Am* 2004;35:43-56.

18. Sengputa D, Senegas J: Mechanical supplementation by non-rigid fixation in degenerative intervertebral lumbar segments: The Wallis System. *Eur Spine J* 2002;11(suppl):164-169.

19. Mulholland R, Sengupta D: Rationale, principles and experimental evaluation of the concept of soft tissue stabilization. *Eur Spine J* 2002;11(suppl):198-205.

20. Hadlow S, Fagan A, Hillier T, Fraser R: The Graf ligamentoplasty procedure: Comparison with posterolateral fusion in the management of low back pain. *Spine* 1998;23:1172-1179.

21. Gardner A, Pande K: Graf ligamentoplasty: A 7 year follow-up. *Eur Spine J* 2002;11(suppl):157-163.

22. Brechnbuhler D, Markwalder T, Braun M: Surgical results after soft tissue stabilization of the lumbar spine in degenerative disc disease: Long-term results. *Acta Neurochir* 1998;140:521-525.

23. Hashimoto T, Oha F, Shigenobu K, et al: Mid-term clinical results of Graf stabilization for lumbar degenerative pathologies: A minimum 2-year follow-up. *Spine J* 2001;1:283-289.

24. Stoll T, Dubois G, Schwarzenbach O: The Dynamic Neutralization System for the spine: A multicenter study of a novel non-fusion system. *Eur Spine J* 2002;11(suppl):170-178.

25. Fernstrom U: Arthroplasty with Intercorporal Endoprosthesis in herniated disc and in painful disc. *Acta Chir Scand* 1966;357(suppl):154-159.

26. Sagi H, Bao Q, Yuan H: Nuclear replacement strategies. *Orthop Clin North Am* 2003;34:263-267.

27. Bertagnoli R, Schonmayr R: Surgical and clinical results with the PDN Prosthetic Disc-Nucleus Device. *Eur Spine J* 2002;11(suppl):143-148.

28. Klara P, Ray C: Artificial nucleus replacement: Clinical experience. *Spine* 2002;27:1374-1377.

29. Enker P, Steffee A, McMillin C, et al: Artificial disc replacement: Preliminary report with a 3-year minimum follow-up. *Spine* 1983;18:1061-1070.

30. Griffith S, Shelokov A, Buttner-Janz K, et al: A multicenter retrospective study of the clinical results of the LINK SB Charite Intervertebral Prosthesis: The initial European experience. *Spine* 1994;19:1842-1849.

31. de Kleuver M, Oner F, Jacobs W: Total disc replacement for chronic low back pain: Background systematic review of the literature. *Eur Spine J* 2003;12:108-116.

32. Hochshuler S, Ohnmeiss D, Guyer R, et al: Artificial disc: Preliminary results of a prospective study in the United States. *Eur Spine J* 2002;11(suppl):106-110.

33. Blumenthal S, Ohnmeiss D, Guyer R, Hochshuler S: Prospective study evaluating total disc replacement: Preliminary results. *J Spinal Disord Tech* 2003;16:450-454.

34. Guyer R, McAfee P, Hochschuler S, et al: Prospective randomized study of the Charite artificial disc: Data from two investigational centers. *Spine J* 2004;4(suppl):252S-259S.

35. Cunningham BW, Gordon J, Dmitriev A, Hu N, McAfee P: Biomechanical evaluation of total disc replacement arthroplasty: An in vitro human cadaveric model. *Spine* 2003;28(suppl):S110-S117.

36. Zigler J, Burd T, Vialle E, et al: Lumbar spine arthroplasty: Early results using the ProDisc II. A prospective randomized trial of arthroplasty versus fusion. *J Spinal Disord Tech* 2003;16:369-383.

37. Zigler J: Lumbar spine arthroplasty using the ProDisc II. *Spine J* 2004;4:260S-267S.

38. Delamarter RB, Fribourg DM, Kanim LE, Bae H: ProDisc artificial total lumbar disc replacement: Introduction and early results from the United States clinical trial. *Spine* 2003;28(suppl):S167-S175.

INDEX